Bronte Cullis lived in Canada for five years trying to recover from anorexia nervosa. A gifted artist, Bronte has completed an interior design and make-up design course since returning to her home city of Melbourne. She plans to establish a career in the art world. This is her first book.

Steve Bibb is a successful television producer who owns his own company, Flyscreen Productions. Steve met Bronte Cullis while working with Ray Martin for the Nine Network Australia in 1999. Since then he has produced and directed two one-hour documentaries on Bronte, her mother Jan and their efforts to help eating disorder sufferers. This is his first book.

Bronte's Story

Bronte's Story

Tears, Trials and Triumphs:
A Personal Battle with Anorexia

Bronte Cullis and Steve Bibb

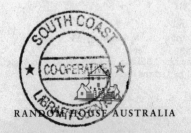

RANDOM HOUSE AUSTRALIA

Random House Australia Pty Ltd
Level 3, 100 Pacific Highway, North Sydney, NSW 2060
http://www.randomhouse.com.au

Sydney   New York   Toronto
London   Auckland   Johannesburg

First published by Random House Australia 2004

National Library of Australia
Cataloguing-in-Publication Entry

Bibb, Steven.
  Bronte's story – tears, trials and triumphs: a personal battle with anorexia.

  ISBN 978 1 74051 307 4.
  ISBN 1 74051 307 X.

  1. Cullis, Bronte. 2. Anorexia nervosa – Patients – Victoria –
  Melbourne – Biography. 3. Eating disorders in adolescence.
  I. Title.

  616.852620092

Cover design by Darian Causby/Highway 51
Cover photograph by Gilly Bibb
Typeset and designed by Midland Typesetters, Maryborough, Victoria
Printed and bound by Griffin Press, South Australia

15 14 13 12 11

For my dad, my unsung hero.
Bronte

For my wife, Gilly.
Steve

Contents

A Note From Bronte

I never thought I would write a book. In fact, much like my appearances on television, this book is something I didn't plan on doing or even want to do. Somehow it just came about. I am so grateful to be given the opportunity to share my story – raw yet cathartic as it has been to relive the past – because I hope I can shed some light of understanding and truth about anorexia nervosa, the condition, my 'head', the negative mind and finally 'Neg', as I have come to know it.

I use all of the above terms throughout the book to describe the same thing – my anorexia. I do this not to confuse you, but rather to show you the level of understanding I had of my illness throughout the process of my recovery. At each stage it was referred to as something different. It has only been since my anorexia was pegged as 'Neg' that I have been truly able to see it for what it is.

This book, my words of truth, would not have been possible without an amazing group of people around me. To my Mum and Dad, you have taught me the true meaning of unconditional love. I wouldn't be here today without that love and your dedication and sacrifices. I am who I am because of you. I adore you both. To my siblings, Samantha, Jordan and James, without the sacrifices you so generously made for me, our family would not have made it. Thank you for your constant support. I am in your debt forever. I love you all beyond words. To all the people at the Bronte Foundation, thank you for inspiring me every day.

Thanks go to my co-author Steve Bibb. Without you, Bibby, this would not have been possible. Thank you for caring, thank you for learning and thank you for understanding. Your written cherries, knowledge and wisdom were truly invaluable. I can't forget to thank Charlie Bibb for lending me his space and Gilly Bibb for her exceptional hospitality also. You have all made the journey so much more enjoyable and rich. I cherish your friendship.

To my Aunty Bronte and Uncle Bryan, I thank you for your many forms of support over the years. I know I wouldn't be here without your help. My thanks also go to my publisher Jeanne Ryckmans, editor Jody Lee, project editor Lydia Papandrea and all at Random House Australia for believing and taking a chance on me.

To Ray Martin and Channel Nine, thank you for giving me the opportunity to share my story and reach the Australian community. Which brings me to my last 'thank you'. To the Australian public, thank you. You have bestowed such kindness, love and support on my family and me. Never lose the spirit that I have seen and have been touched by. It makes the world so much brighter. May you know that I wouldn't be here, and none of this would be possible, this story is not complete without you.

Finally, to all those out there who are in the grips of an eating disorder, whether sufferer, family or friend, I plead with you to live for hope. This is a story of hope. It is real, honest, painful and triumphant. I am here to tell you that life is worth the long fight.

Bronte Cullis

A Note From Steve

This is an odd book. Neither Bronte nor I pretend to be authors in the true literary sense. What we hope to be are storytellers. *Bronte's Story* is red raw, painful and honest – a real life story of survival from a baffling illness. This book is based on Bronte's diaries from 1994 until 2000 as she spiralled into anorexia's clutches before somehow escaping death. Ultimately, this is a book of hope.

When we started out on this book, I knew we had a great story and a strong foundation in the diaries. I also knew Bronte had a profile thanks to the television shows I have produced over the years. What I didn't realise was the depth and extent of Bronte's story. During the hours of interviews I conducted for this book, I was amazed at what happened behind the scenes in the Cullis family. How can anyone, or any family, survive this torment? Anorexia nervosa, as I have now discovered, shocks you to the core. I have shed a few tears for the sufferers and their families I have met.

This book became more than a diary. It's a collection of anecdotes, moments, observations, recollections and encounters. Above all, I hope it will touch your heart and give hope to all the people, and their families, suffering today. I also hope readers will understand that the term, 'eating disorder', is a misnomer. In truth, it is a disgusting disease of the mind.

I walked into Bronte Cullis' tortured life under a brightly lit Christmas tree in the lobby of a Canadian hotel in 1999. I was producing a prime-time special for the Nine Network, which I called *Bronte's Story*. The title seems to have stuck. Since that first encounter, I have got to know a wonderful person in Bronte Cullis. I'm proud to call her a friend and I'm honoured to know that the feeling is mutual.

I want to thank several people for getting this book out of our brains and into your hands. Firstly, to Jan and Graeme Cullis for trusting me and for their invaluable input. You are both wonderful people. To Samantha, Jordan and James for supporting Bronte. To Jeanne Ryckmans, our publisher, who convinced all at Random House this book was worth a shot. To Jody Lee, our editor, and Lydia Papandrea, our project editor for their patience, talent and drive to improve. To Ray Martin, for writing the foreword, for being a mate and for introducing me to Bronte while we worked together on *A Current Affair*. Thanks also to Deborah Munro for transcribing Bronte's diaries and to Claire Harris for having the patience to transcribe my rambling interviews. I'd also like to thank Margie Bashfield, Joe Ferma and Mick Morris for their sharp memories. Also, a huge thanks to Robyn Lowe and Anne Reilly for their advice.

Finally, and most importantly, to my family. To my wife Gilly, my best friend and the love of my life, thank you for your constant love, endless patience and for feeding Bronte and me during the writing of this book while you were heavily pregnant. To my son Charlie for letting Bronte use his bedroom, and to my second son, Archie, for being born on the day this book was finished.

Steve Bibb

Foreword

Through the looking glass, living with Bronte must have been a crazy kaleidoscope for Jan and Graeme Cullis. Yet, there was no life without her. Jan said that to me many times. That's why they never gave up when everybody else did.

Now Bronte's demons have been tamed – she's still got all the rich colours, just missing the madness.

Lean on me, when you're not strong . . .

When the karaoke lights up for a chorus or two, anybody can be somebody, just follow the bouncing ball. Bronte was just being Bronte. Up there on stage in a Brisbane pub the other Saturday night, wearing white-cotton hipsters and an egg-shell blue shirt, belting out the old Bill Withers' classic.

This Saturday night, it's Bronte unplugged – on parade, singing and laughing. Laughing in the spotlight, a winner for all the world to see. Tonight, the sparkling queen of pop, yesterday the princess of eating disorders.

Send in the clowns.

For too many years, Bronte shuffled along life's foot-path with her head down and her shoulders hunched – apologising for just being alive. Back then, the only Saturday night fever she knew was a frantic race to the hospital emergency ward.

On this happy night her dad was a lonely bystander,

lost in the karaoke crowd. While I watched him, he watched her. Graeme's eternally and paternally proud of Bronte − as he should be. I saw him steal a selfish grin. He'd done the hard yards and had every right to be selfish. After all, he'd helped save her life.

Every picture in Graeme's memory is worth a thousand tears.

Like when Bronte screamed in his face and told him she hated him. I remember he just smiled and told her that he loved her. And he surely did. He knew this wasn't Bronte screaming. He knew she really adored him. And she does. They're great mates again.

What a painful, emotional journey it's been for the Cullis clan − to hell and back.

On the stairs, above the karaoke carousel, Jan stands watch, as she always has. Like Graeme, I suspect Jan is remembering another lifetime, too. A very different existence. Bronte the life of the party? Bronte the chanteuse? Tell her she's dreaming.

Could this be the same shy, twisted waif they carted off to the much-maligned Canadian clinic, to help her somehow locate the life she'd lost? They found it, hiding deep down in her brittle bones.

Bronte's mum is one of the most remarkable women I've come across. Strong, good tempered and full of unrequited compassion. Not just for Bronte but for anybody who's hurting. She's what you'd call 'a good woman'.

Jan has turned the agony and ecstasy of the last decade into a university thesis. Dr Cullis, I presume. Anorexia, bulimia and all that jazz.

Forget reality television. The Cullis family saga is real life melodrama. It's an incredible yarn. Truth, weirder than fiction − and much more fun.

In telling Bronte's story, I must admit my bias. I think 'Miss B', as I affectionately call her, is simply special. I hope you will, too.

Ray Martin

Prologue

My name is Bronte Cullis. I'm twenty-five years old and I shouldn't be writing these words to you. I should have died, several years ago, a slow and painful death. For most of my life I've been gripped by a terrible demon in my mind, which is called anorexia nervosa. It is a vile mental disease that is as deadly as it is strange. Somehow I survived to tell the story you are about to read – my story.

I was about ten years old when the first signs of this monster called anorexia started to simmer to the surface – not that my family and I realised it at the time. I would hide under our house for hours on end trying to figure out why I had such dark and evil thoughts in my head. While I found the rough dirt floor, the cool air and the darkness strangely soothing, they did not help me shake the awful things I was thinking about myself. I didn't want to tell anyone about the thoughts in case they suspected I was crazy. What then? What if I was crazy? So I kept the thoughts to myself, which was the worst thing I could have done, but how was I to know?

I stopped eating completely the day my Nanny was diagnosed with a tumour. It was the final trigger needed by my anorexia, which suddenly leapt for joy and got to work. Outwardly, I denied I had a problem but deep inside I was being tortured. There seemed no way out.

I didn't mean to begin starving myself to death but that's what happened.

At the age of fifteen, I was admitted to hospital for the first time. My weight was terrifyingly low but not my lowest weight, as it turned out. That was to come. To stay alive, I was fed liquid supplements through a long tube that was run up my nose and down into my stomach. It's called a nasogastric tube and is even more painful than it sounds. To most people I looked like I was about to die.

The doctors really didn't know how to treat my anorexia. They simply fed me through the tube, got my weight up and sent me back into the world I hated. They didn't treat the mental illness and I quickly spiralled backwards and close to death in the emergency ward again and again. There was nothing my parents or doctors could say, or do, to save me.

My family and I were told by several experts I was the worst case of anorexia they had ever seen. Some doctors even told my parents to give up trying to save my life as I was going to die anyway. My last chance was a controversial clinic on the other side of the world that caused me a great deal of pain and suffering with the aim of curing me.

It has been an awful journey to hell and back, but I have made it. This is my story. It is a story of hope.

Part One

The Mansion

It was called 'The Mansion'. A grand old Canadian home, imposing you could say, clad in neat, white weatherboards and slate-grey shingles. The windows looked like tired eyes, their black frames like bags under your eyes the morning after a big night out. The roof had been recently restored and was now a bright terracotta red, which was in stark contrast to the lived-in look of the rest of the house. The steps leading up to the wooden front door were painted black but now in desperate need of another coat, such was the foot traffic over the years. The Mansion was in a pretty little town called Victoria on Vancouver Island. As we walked up those steps to the front door, my heart sank and I didn't want to go inside. I was terrified. This was Montreux, my so-called salvation and my future. I stood still, squeezing the life out of my Mum and Dad's hands, wishing I could vanish into thin air.

The Montreux Counselling Centre was controversial and so was its founder, Peggy Claude-Pierre. A strong-willed Canadian, Peggy founded the clinic in 1988 on the strength of her studies and the lessons she learned nursing her two anorexic daughters, Kirsten and Nicole, back to health. Patients lived at Montreux to receive 24-hour care. It was a clinic that cared for the sufferers of anorexia and bulimia considered beyond help – the hopeless ones left to die by the world's medical systems.

This little clinic quickly became famous and grew quite large. With fame came controversy over Montreux's holistic approach, treatment methods, high cost, and self claims of almost 100 per cent recovery. It was clear that Peggy and the clinic annoyed some in the medical establishment. Most of the workers were not medical practitioners – although all patients were medically monitored – and many of these workers were former anorexics and bulimics. Where traditional hospitals punished anorexics, Peggy offered love, self-esteem and hope. Controversy aside, this was it. My last chance at life.

Noah, one of the managers at Montreux, greeted us with a smile and ushered us into the lobby. Where I expected light inside, everything was dark. There was dark timber panelling on the walls, dark timber floorboards, dark timber doors and a dark timber staircase and balustrade leading into an unknown world that I was unwillingly about to join. The only natural light source was the timid rays of Canadian sunshine seeping through the stained-glass window above the staircase. It was not enough to properly light the space; that job was left to the soft yellow glow of the period table lamps scattered around the rooms. There was a certain smell too, but I don't know that I can describe what it was. It was just an odd smell. There was an eerie aura about this place made more dramatic by opera music gently tiptoeing its way through the half light. This place was not like I had imagined it would be.

Even though it was fairly dark, there was still enough light for me to notice the bags of groceries sitting on the lobby floor. The sudden sight of food scared the life out of me and I began to panic. Noah, the quirky red-headed former Canadian rollerskating champion, was the first to react and rushed me away from the groceries and into his office. My parents and my younger brother James were taken in the opposite direction to meet the administration staff. Noah was trying to quickly calm me by making conversation but all I wanted to do was turn around and run for home. In a desperate attempt to break the ice, Noah said, 'How does it feel to leave Victoria to come to Victoria?' His effort to lighten the moment, well meaning as it was, didn't help. I was in no mood for humour.

Eventually the groceries were taken away and Noah calmed me down enough for me to rejoin Mum and Dad in a larger room next to the lobby. The conference room was never really used for conferences, I don't really know how it got its name. It must have been the living room or a parlour at one time for a wealthy family. Now it was quite sparse and uninviting. A tired oriental rug lay in the middle of the floor and green corduroy sofas and arm-chairs were littered around the edge of the room. There was a fireplace that didn't work and French doors at the far end of the room that didn't open. It was in this cold, strange room that my devoted parents, Jan and Graeme Cullis, left me in the care of complete strangers on 1 May 1996. I sat there begging my parents not to leave me. They did and I cried my heart out.

My parents stayed near Montreux for ten days. I was tired and cold the last day I met them in the conference room. I told them how much I hated being at Montreux and that I wanted to leave. Mum found a handmade teddy bear downtown that looked just like our dog, Muffin. She told me to hold on tight to her and that she would keep me safe. I didn't just cry when they left, for good this time. I wept uncontrollably. I clung on to Dad with both my arms around his neck and would not let go. A clinic worker had to drag me away so my parents could leave. I was held down, screaming, as my parents drove away. I was all on my own and I didn't know if I would ever see them again. This was my last chance at life and I was without my family. The thought just about killed me.

Part Two

Childhood

Mum knew something was terribly wrong when she was about to give birth to me. She didn't quite know what it was or how to explain it to the nurses, she just sensed that I was in big trouble. It was 3 January 1979. I was ten days overdue. By 11 a.m. that day, the nurses and doctor also realised I was in trouble and something drastic needed to be done. With no time for an emergency Caesarean section, Mum was strapped to the delivery table and Dad was ordered out of the room. Out came the forceps. The next 45 minutes were the longest and most painful in Mum's life. Without pain management or sedation, Mum had a high forceps extraction that caused severe damage to my head. I was eventually delivered just before midday.

I weighed 7 lb and 15 ounces when I was born. I had a huge fracture on the top of my skull caused by the forceps. No one was sure if I would live.

While I fought for my brief life, Mum lay exhausted in her hospital bed. A few days later, a stern-looking woman walked up to Mum and introduced herself as Australia's only female paediatric neurosurgeon. Mum was understandably relieved because here was the doctor who would fix my skull. Mum's optimism soon evaporated when the doctor said I needed surgery because I would die without it. The news got worse. There was a chance, the neurosurgeon said, that I could die during – or after – surgery. There was also a chance I could end up in a vegetative state. To cap it off, Mum was told that the technique of elevating the skull of a newborn was risky. It had only been performed on two babies before me. The next day, a week after I was born, I went under the knife.

The operation took three hours. The surgeon likened the procedure to drilling a hole in a dented ping-pong ball and gently pulling back on the dent to restore its perfect shape. I emerged from surgery looking battle-scarred with a huge, angry-looking arc across my skull. 'Don't press here' was written on masking tape torn from a roll and stuck just above the surgeon's incision. Mum said I cried for weeks.

I was allowed to go home one month after the opera-tion. Five months later, Mum's appendix, ironically the source of pain throughout her pregnancy, finally burst one Saturday evening. She was admitted to hospital and underwent an emergency appendectomy. Suddenly my Mum was ripped away from me and, in response, I stop-ped eating. After six days, I was weak with hunger. Mum managed to feed me from a bottle when I fell asleep. It became the way I ate from that day on.

When I was born, our family – Mum, Dad, my sister Samantha and brother Jordan – lived at Safety Beach, a suburb on the wonderful Mornington Peninsula in Port Phillip Bay. Home was an old holiday house that Dad bought from his father. It was a funny little shack. Dad's father and grandfather built it themselves using mainly leftover train carriage parts from when Dad's grandfather worked as a carriage builder for Victorian railways. Out the back was a small flat and an outdoor shower to rinse off the salt water after swimming. We lived one street back from the beach and for six weeks of the year Safety Beach was crowded. The rest of the time it was a lonely place for Mum. She was a stay at home mum with three children under five. Dad worked long hours as a survey draughtsman for the Westernport Bay Planning Authority.

By the time I was about three years old the family had moved twice because Dad changed jobs and needed to be closer to his work. Baby James had also joined the family. Our first move was from the Mornington Peninsula to a potato farm in country Victoria for a few years before shifting to the old gold-mining town of Garfield in the Gippsland District. Dad was a bus driver and had to commute all the way into Melbourne. We lived on a quarter-acre block in Garfield surrounded by dairy cattle, orchards and more potato farms. It had all the makings of a perfect life. We had a red setter, Molly, plus a menagerie of pets – chickens, cows, dogs, cats, rabbits and budgies. The budgies all lived in our sunroom except one called Charlie who had the run of the brick-veneer house because he could dance, sing and chat like a true member of the Cullis family. That was until Spot the cat ate Charlie the budgie.

Every Christmas we would go camping at Corowa on the New South Wales border. On these trips the Cullis kids would canoe down the mighty Murray River while being eaten alive by mosquitoes. We would then find the biggest and best gum tree to perform human bombs into the murky waters. Trips like these were simply blissful, as were our Christmas mornings when we would wake up at some insane hour and excitedly chatter until it was light enough to wake Mum and Dad. These memories fill

my soul with such brightness. Life was pure and simple.
We were best friends and we were happy.

Despite my shaky start in life, I became physically
stronger until one day I ended up in hospital – once again
fighting for my life.

Our idyll was shattered on the first day at school for my
older brother Jordan. I was almost three and my brother
James was just six months old. Mum had dropped
Jordan off at school and was heading into Garfield to run
a few errands. She parked the car in the main street and
unloaded me and put baby James in his pram. We crossed
the street and headed towards the post office. Suddenly,
Mum realised she'd left her wallet on the front seat of
the car. Without thinking, she walked back to the car.
As she was about to touch the door, she remembered she
hadn't told me to wait on the footpath with James. As
she turned around she saw a yellow Volvo sedan hit me
and throw me 10 metres down the road. The Volvo driver
was kneeling over me and praying by the time Mum had
sprinted across the street.

It took the ambulance 50 minutes to reach the nearest
hospital, Dandenong. I had a broken thighbone, a broken right arm and had fractured my skull again. It was
the final injury that brought a smile to the doctor's face.
It turned out that my extra thick skull, the result of the
neurosurgery, had almost certainly saved my life because
it's where the Volvo's bumper bar struck me.

After three months of traction I said goodbye to the
hospital and hello to family life once again. By now I was
especially close to Jordan. He would always get me into
some sort of trouble. He was a non-stop kid who dragged

me along on his adventures. One morning, Jordan decided he would take me swimming in the drain that ran past our nature strip. I was still under doctor's orders not to walk because my break was still healing and any strain could mean a second break. Determined to forge ahead with the adventure of the day, Jordan found two tennis rackets, turned them upside down and got me to use them as substitute crutches. We could have drowned in that drain. It was only by a stroke of luck that Jordan spotted a snake in the water and decided to take me back to the house only to find Mum frantically searching for us. Jordan was such an inquisitive kid that even under lock and key he would somehow escape to discover a new adventure. He was the instigator of all things 'naughty' in our house.

I've always been a little eccentric at times but as I became more sick certain behaviours and my fears turned into deep obsessions. I became obsessive-compulsive about most things. When I was about seven I started having nightmares that the latest tragedy, illness or way to die plastered on the news would happen to my family and me. So in the mid-1980s when AIDS became the world's latest misunderstood disease, my negative mind made it the central fear of my nightmares. After this, the nightmares always remained the same. My fear grew and grew until it was so huge that it teamed up with my anorexia to control me through a destructive series of rituals.

At the age of eight, it was time to change schools when Mum and Dad decided to leave country life behind and moved to the outskirts of Melbourne; to a new sprawling suburb called Rowville. We lived with Mum's parents for many months while we looked for a house to rent. Not long after we found a house, Mum and Dad took the opportunity to build a new house on a recently opened housing estate on the other side of Rowville. While this was being built, we stayed with Dad's parents for about a year – all four siblings in Dad's old childhood bedroom. Finally, the new house was finished and we moved.

It was under the new house in Rowville that I started to escape from reality by retreating into the safety of my own space, my own private world. My secret world was made up of a cool dirt floor, red brick foundations, hardwood timber beams and the undersides of Cypress pine floorboards. The only light was provided by the occasional rays of sunshine poking through the gaps in the mortar of the brickwork. I decorated my hideaway with picnic rugs and ate passionfruit from a vine that grew in the sunshine on the outside. For company I recruited our pet dog Tiger, an American cocker spaniel.

I've always had deep, dark 'thoughts' but I remember them becoming a big problem when I was nine years old. The thoughts didn't start out as a voice; they became more voice-like as time went by. The thoughts became larger, louder and more continuous until they became a dominant male-like voice constantly telling me I wasn't worthy of life. It was a singular voice but it didn't have a tone like a particular voice and it certainly wasn't another personality.

I was too afraid to tell people about the voice because of what they would think of me. In fact, I'd been too scared to divulge these intimate thoughts my entire life, worried about what the world would think of me. I was afraid that people would think I was crazy. I felt trapped because no matter which way I turned these thoughts were there threatening and convincing me that if I didn't do something Mum, Dad and everyone I loved would be devoured by a crocodile, killed in a car crash or would get AIDS. The last one was the interesting fear. I was so terrified of the disease that I couldn't even bring myself to write or say the word AIDS until I was much older. Even if I did what the voice told me to do I still felt this way. These thoughts would come into my head without even giving me the chance to think about it. Much like instant coffee, these were instant thoughts.

It's amazing how fear can cloud your ability to think logically and cause you to act in a phobic way. The fears that teamed up with my negative mind eventually became everyday thoughts and feelings. They became so black and brutal that eventually it became like a single voice. It used my fears and turned them into realities for me. It was a bully and a dictator. This is perhaps why I described it as a voice.

By ten I would hide under the house whenever someone was angry or sad. I thought that everything bad in the world was somehow my fault.

My parents worked hard to give all four Cullis children the best education and life experiences. At the time, they were busy and I was a very quiet child who did everything I was supposed to do. This meant I could easily fade away into the background of a busy family. My Dad hardly noticed I was alive because I didn't play basketball

– his passion – and I didn't do anything that interested him. He, like everyone else, thought I was happy doing my own thing so he left me to my own devices. I felt I was in the way most of the time, which is why I wanted to disappear. It wasn't that I didn't love my family, I adored them. I truly thought their lives would be better without me.

No one ever came to rescue me in my private world. I just sat under the house for hours quietly thinking about my sad life, all the time making myself feel worse. I would plot ways of running away so I wouldn't be in anyone's road. I also wanted to escape from myself. Part of me just wanted to die so I wouldn't have to think about how bad I was and how much space I was wasting.

I would also think the world was such a useless place because there were so many bad things going on. I was watching the television news one day when they were explaining how a train hit and killed someone. I just sat there thinking, 'This is all it ever is. There's nothing good.'

This basket full of fears kept me from ever really trusting life. From the age of ten, I would patrol the house after everyone had gone to bed, like a security guard on the night watch. Firstly, I would check every window and door to make sure they were locked. Then I would move on to the appliances and switch off the power at the wall. My safety rounds done, I would check that everyone was breathing. I'd stand right next to every family member and listen for the sound of their breath and watch for the rise of their chests. Luckily my Dad snored so I would always know he was alive. Sometimes during summer Mum or Dad would get up later in the night and open a window to let in a cool breeze. I would sense that a window was open and wake to do a second round of the house until I found the offending window and closed it. Job done and house safe, Bronte Cullis, security guard, would go back to bed.

One night I was woken by strange noises coming from my brothers' room. I got up and crept around the corner to see into the room. It was dark and I couldn't see much but I could make out a shadowy figure. I had no weapon (good security guard!) and I started to panic. I was sure we were all about to die so I ran to Mum and Dad's room as fast as I could, manoeuvring my way around the furniture in the dark, and woke them with the dreadful news of the intruder. Dad led me to the bedroom and very boldly switched on the light to find my little brother James sitting on the ground playing with his Lego set!

Emergency sirens would also set me off. Whenever I was home alone I would instantly panic at the sound of a siren. I was convinced the ambulance was racing to an accident where a family member had been killed. Dread would completely envelop me to the point that I would be in tears, ready to check the hospitals. Then the family would come home, just as safely as they had left.

I've always felt the need to be at home to protect my family so I didn't do the typical things such as slumber parties at a friend's house. If I wasn't at home who would protect my family from the mass murderers out there? Who would stop the house burning down and who would save those trapped inside? The only other place I felt safe was at my Nanny and Poppa's house yet I still had sleepless and stressful nights worrying about my home and my family. These were terrifying thoughts for such a little person. I would leave 'I love you' notes on Mum and Dad's pillows in the mornings before I went to school. My fear was that if I didn't do this something would happen to them during the day and they would never know how much I loved them. They didn't understand why I was doing it. They didn't know I had these fears cascading around in my head. As I mentioned, I didn't tell anyone because I was worried they might think I was crazy. I was a kid and I was confused. When Dad told me to stop leaving the notes I was sure my family hated me and didn't want me around.

When I come across a child behaving like an angel now, I worry. I was never once disciplined or smacked by my parents because I never put a foot out of line. Household duty meetings were held on Sundays in our house. I lived with three 'normal' children who were sometimes naughty, messy and lazy when it came to chores. I must have been about ten when Mum would take up these issues with all the children but all I heard was, 'Bronte, the house isn't clean enough, why are you so messy and lazy?' I would take it all onboard and I would then proceed to wash, scrub, clean and iron until a few weeks later the same issues would be raised with the 'children'. I would berate myself for not doing a good enough job the first time. All I wanted to do was make my Mum happy and it seemed I was failing miserably.

I took everything so personally as a child. I felt everyone was always laughing at me and thinking I was stupid. I remember one time shouting out, 'Look Dad, there's the Waverley Munchpickle (municipal) golf course!' It brought a round of laughter which, to me, meant that I was laughable. Frightened of failure, I stopped speaking in public and began to withdraw from anything involving social activities. Life had, quite simply, become too risky. Failure and not fitting in lurked around every corner.

When I was a little girl, I used to go to Sunday School where we were taught that Sunday was a day of rest. Unlike most children I took this message very seriously. Things got pretty bad when Mum and Dad took James and I swimming at the local council pool after Sunday School. They obviously chose Sunday because they both worked six days a week and this was the most convenient time. But I was emotionally torn because of the thoughts in my head telling me that God would infect Mum and Dad with AIDS because we should be resting.

One Sunday I was so stressed out about what was going to happen that I started pacing around the outside of the house. Dad was sitting inside and saw me pass the window a couple of times. Worried, he came out to ask what was wrong and why I was doing laps of the house. I was crying and could barely speak. I eventually calmed down enough to tell him why I was so distressed. It was the first time I told anyone that I had these bizarre thoughts in my head.

Being considered weird was one thing but exposing myself as possibly being officially crazy was something else all together. Dad's response was simple and to the point. 'Don't be silly. We can't possibly have AIDS. Swimming in the local pool isn't how you get AIDS.' His clear logic was wasted on my illogical fear and simply made me feel stupid. The more people told me 'don't be silly', the more I thought I was different, crazy and stupid. Telling Mum and Dad didn't ease the pain of the voice and its commands as I'd hoped. It actually became worse . . . and it was about to get a lot worse.

About the same time I became paranoid of being in public places because I was convinced that I would somehow catch AIDS, and when I did venture out for a walk, I would stare at the ground to make sure I didn't step on food or syringes. I heard a story when I was younger about someone being pricked with a needle on public transport. The thought terrified me so whenever I had to sit in public places Dad would repeatedly slap the seat and run his hand over it to prove there were no hidden needles.

One day, a few years later on a trip to Sydney, Dad and I caught the Manly ferry to take in some sights. There was no way I was going to sit down so Dad started frantically hitting the seats to prove they were safe. It was quite a crowded ferry. I can't imagine what the other passengers must have thought as this crazy man went around banging seats while a sick-looking skinny girl screamed in horror. At the time, to me and my negative mind's fears and obsessions, this sort of thing almost seemed normal.

Given the chance, I would never want to go through childhood again. When I'm asked if I had a good childhood I say it was sad. Not because of my family or external things but because of myself. Unfortunately my parents didn't understand me then and I kept all my thoughts – my internal hatred – to myself. My parents didn't know what was going on inside that little blonde head of mine. People thought I was weird and I felt as if I was indeed weird. Seeing how different my behaviours and emotions were to everyone else, I decided to keep it all to myself. Besides, I didn't want to burden my family with my pain – I figured they had their own problems.

There was always some sort of drama going on in the Cullis family, usually involving hospitals. One incident that sums up what it was like happened when I was sixteen. I was in the Monash Medical Centre being treated for anorexia and my sister Samantha was in the same hospital recovering from surgery to remover a tumour on her thyroid. Dad stayed at home with James while Mum visited Sam and me. When she finally got home, Mum found an empty house. The covers of both Dad and James' beds were thrown back and were still warm. As Mum started to panic the phone rang. It was Dad. James had broken his arm falling off the top bunk bed and was now in Monash Hospital. Three Cullis children all in the same hospital. To top it off, a friend called later the same night to say my older brother Jordan was also in Monash Hospital – this time in Emergency – with a broken ankle. The injury happened 40 kilometres away but Jordan's friend decided to drive him all the way across town for treatment. When asked why, he said he thought my parents would want their children all in the one place. Very thoughtful.

1994

Sunday, 3 July 1994

It's more than halfway through the year and this is the first time I've written in my diary which is a sin – a terrible sin. I sometimes wonder what kind of person I am. Am I good or am I bad? Am I just an average being with no talents? Sometimes I really feel like I don't know myself.

I'm halfway through Year 10 at school and I'm very confused about absolutely everything. I'm so sick of having to act happy on the outside. Sometimes, I feel my parents just aren't interested in what I do! My Nanny, however, is always there for me and is always supporting me. I don't want to go into great detail but let me just say she has been pretty sick lately with a tumour on her face and we thought she was going to die. I hate that word! I was so scared! I just couldn't imagine Nanny not being here with me everyday of my life. She plays such a big part in my life. I wish she could live forever.

Anorexia stole time from significant people in my life, one being my Nanny. Patricia Eastwood Clarke was born eight weeks prematurely in 1927 and was placed in a shoebox, wrapped in cotton wool and put beside a sunny window to help her fight for her life. I guess she was given little chance of living.

At the age of eight, Nanny was hit by a truck while riding her scooter down Canterbury Road in Melbourne's Surrey Hills. She suffered damage to the brain but, being the trooper she is, survived. Traumatic birth, car accidents; there are many parallels between our lives which is why we've always been soul mates. Nanny sat beside me while I recovered from neurosurgery and she sat with me in the hospital after I was hit by the Volvo. She called me her 'clinging little vine' when I was young. If I wasn't with my Mum, you could find me clinging to Nanny's leg.

As I grew up, Nanny became one of my best friends. She accepted and loved me unconditionally. I have many wonderful childhood memories of holidays with my Nanny and Poppa, John Patrick Clarke, driving all over the countryside and exploring the city of Melbourne. Nanny would take me everywhere with her. I would tag along and help her deliver meals on wheels and we would volunteer at Villa Maria Society for the Blind. She has always given herself to the community, which is where my love for volunteer work was born. She has always been far fitter than me. She would take me bike riding and she would always be miles ahead of me.

My Nanny and Poppa were always travelling so when an opportunity came along for them to teach English to Cambodian refugees in Thailand they jumped at it. They were gone for two years and I was devastated. When they returned we discovered they had arranged to sponsor quite a few refugee families to live in Australia. A few years later I was involved with another one of my Poppa's generous gestures when he organised for a group of Chernobyl children to stay with them while they were holidaying from Russia. They all had cancer. We took them to the Royal Melbourne Show. They couldn't speak a word of English and we couldn't speak a word of Russian but it was one of the most moving experiences of my life. This was life with my grandparents – surprises around every corner, living life to the full, bestowing kindness on others, loving everyone and loving each other.

I loved my Poppa. He was one of thirteen brothers and grew up in suburban Melbourne. He met Nanny at a dance one night. They fell in love and married. He was hilarious, eccentric, wonderfully passionate and very alive. *Fatal Attraction* was his favourite movie! He was a dreamer while Nanny was the stable one, the hard worker. Over the years, this former army cook turned his hand to just about anything. He was a painter, a window-washer, ran a milkbar and a pet food business. They moved to Adelaide to raise their six children – one being my Mum, Jan. His passion lives on in us. He was the instigator of the Friday night lolly party throughout my childhood and instilled in me the love of lollies. It was my refusal of one of Poppa's lollies that aroused suspicion of anorexia.

I adore all my grandparents – Dad's parents, Nanna Lorna Clara Hadden and Poppa Herbert George Cullis, are the most wonderful people. But there's something special about Nanny, which is one of the reasons why her illness triggered mine and it is also one of the reasons she too suffered greatly at the hands of my anorexia. The problem was that she loved me and I didn't want any-one to love me so I pushed her away. I became nasty and hostile towards her and the more she would try to help, the more frustrated and angry I would become. Despite my behaviour, she never once let me succeed in my attempts to sabotage my relationship with her. She came almost every day and sat beside my bed at the Monash Medical Centre. She would bring balloons to brighten my room and games and magazines to distract me. No matter how many times I told her to go away, my anorexia told her to go away, she would stay and tell me how much she loved me.

Monday, 4 July 1994

One of my very close friends has just left my school. Her name is Rachel. I'm writing this so I will remember her. I will miss her. It's the second time she has left this year. I don't want her to come back because I know if she does, she will just leave again. I'm so sick of people hurting me. Walking in and out of my life and trampling on my feelings. I'm so sick of being the one on the sideline. I'm afraid to get close to anyone because I think they'll just leave me in a year or two and leave me shattered. I especially hate my school. The teachers only take notice if you're smart. If you're dumb like me then you're nothing.

I'm sick of being nothing. I'm going to make something of myself in this world. I have a place. I just have to find it. I can't believe I just wrote this page of stuff down. I didn't even realise I felt half of this until my pen actually hit the paper.

I often wonder what my niche is in life and if I will ever find it. I just wish I could be good at something like my sister Samantha. She's smart because she's doing medicine at university. She's pretty and is so

looked up to by others. I'm sick of being so inferior and
feeling so inferior. Don't you just hate feelings? Life
would be so much easier without feelings because no
one would get angry with me!

Despite finding it difficult to make true friends at school, there was one special person I could relate to – Rachel. Although we were from very different backgrounds, there was just something we understood about each other. Rachel was very artistic, very intelligent and very misunderstood by others. I suspected she was struggling with her own inner demons at the time when she left school one day and never came back. There was no word of explanation. I remember telling myself that if I was more interesting, a better friend and smarter then Rachel wouldn't have gone. School was already difficult for me and now I had lost what seemed to be the one thing that was good about it. She was the one person I trusted in a place full of typical teenage girls.

Tuesday, 5 July 1994

Dad always seems so angry lately but he's been so
much more relaxed since his holiday started a few
days ago. On Monday, we went for a walk along St
Kilda pier. It was like he had no work stress and he
was really enjoying himself. I liked being around
him. He told us about when he was a kid and how
life has changed from then until now. Next week
we're driving to Adelaide for a holiday, just Mum,
Dad, James and me. I can't wait to spend more
time with Dad. I miss him a lot. I mean I live in the
same house as him but I don't see him all that

much because he works so hard and gets stressed a lot. I wish he could be on holiday all the time.

Wednesday, 6 July 1994

For the past four months I've been on a modelling and deportment course. It's been a lot of fun but I'm getting a bit sick of getting up every Saturday at 8 a.m. to go all the way into the city. Honestly, I don't know how Mum manages it. Every week she takes me in there and spends the day with me. She's a real saint! I sometimes wonder how such good parents ended up with someone like me! I'm very ungrateful and selfish. I really want Mum to know I appreciate everything she has done for me – and I don't want her to think I'm just saying that because I feel obliged to say so! I really am grateful and I really do love her. At least there's one good thing I can say about myself. I have a big heart. Maybe that's why I'm so emotional.

It's the end of another day in beautiful Melbourne. It's a city I love and adore as everyone I love and adore lives here with me. I'll write again tomorrow.

Thursday, 7 July 1994

I absolutely HATE my life. It totally sucks! I'm worthless. Why has my life turned out like this? It's so UNFAIR. I really hate my life and myself. I think my parents consider me a liar, a selfish cow and stupid! I probably am. I amount to nothing.

I can't wait until I move out of home to be who I want to be, do what I want and eat what I want.

I hate myself.

The corn chip gave me away. I thought it was a cunning little ploy. I was using one corn chip as a sort of prop to give the impression I was eating a bowl of nachos with friends at a restaurant. In fact, I didn't eat one chip, or any nachos, all night. I thought no one at the suburban Mexican restaurant noticed my slight of hand. Our group of friends seemed lost in conversation and by the end of the night I was sure that I had flown safely under the radar. I was wrong. One person did notice – my sister Sam.

She didn't confront me until the next morning when she accusingly said, 'You just had the one chip the whole night and played a bit of a magic game, didn't you?' I denied everything, of course. Then Mum started asking why I hadn't eaten the nachos. I told her I had eaten it and that Sam had just been seeing things. My weak answer had 'lie' written all over it. Sam responded with, 'She's sick Mum, I think she has anorexia!' Silence followed. Anorexia? The possibility shocked Mum as she couldn't believe such a thing could be true. But with the evidence stacking up – I had a bout of flu I couldn't shake, I had dropped a noticeable amount of weight and now I had been caught out not eating – she had no choice but to consider that I might be anorexic.

The corn chip episode took place on 4 August 1994 – Sam's nineteenth birthday. Twenty days later I was in hospital. I was fifteen.

To get me to a doctor, Mum pretended I was having my endless flu checked out. I wouldn't have gone any-where near a GP if I knew I was being examined for anorexia. When I got there, the doctor did all the normal check-up things but she also weighed me and ordered blood tests. I started to get angry. I was asked to wait out in reception while Mum stayed back and spoke with the doctor, who told Mum that I definitely had anorexia nervosa.

Mum confronted me that evening in my bedroom. 'You have anorexia,' she said. I denied it and assured her I was fine. A heated argument erupted. I was angry because I didn't think there was anything wrong with me. I'm sure somewhere inside I knew I was sick but I didn't want to deal with, or acknowledge, it. I especially didn't want my family to know. That meant they were noticing me and to be noticed was the last thing I wanted. I wanted to fade away and avoid them saying, 'You've got to eat to become healthy again.'

Every mealtime became a barrage of questions, and a battle, about what I was going to eat. Despite my reassurances to everyone that I was OK, I was taken to see another GP who specialised in eating disorders. I didn't want to see him but I felt my parents would be angry if I didn't go. I liked this GP instantly. He asked me why I couldn't eat. He wasn't angry with me. He just sat there and asked, 'Tell me, why can't you eat?' He seemed gentle and kind. I don't know why I did but I told him how I felt inside. I didn't tell him everything but it was a start.

After the consultation he told my parents that I was too far gone psychologically for him to help and referred me to another doctor, a psychiatrist, which proved to be a complete waste of time. This doctor said I was a controlling child who should just keep quiet and eat up. I saw him for a few weeks and I tried to tell him I wasn't being a brat and I wasn't trying to control everyone. He wouldn't listen so I refused to go back.

I was still managing to attend school at this stage,

although I was also missing chunks of schooling because of all the doctors' appointments. I had to pin my uniforms otherwise they would fall off me.

I remember the first day I blacked out and collapsed at school. I was fifteen and I hadn't eaten breakfast or lunch for days. It was the end of a history lesson and I was sitting on a stool. The classroom was empty apart from Rachel and me. I went to hop down but fainted and crashed to the floor. Rachel ran over, picked me up and revived me with a sip of water. We agreed not to tell anyone what had happened.

The thoughts in my head were telling me not to eat. I would take my lunch to school and pretend to eat it in the schoolyard. When no one was watching I'd throw it into a rubbish bin and quickly shut the lid hoping I wouldn't be caught. No food meant my blood pressure was dropping and I was becoming very weak. Fainting became more common. I didn't tell anyone about these 'turns' because I didn't want anyone to know what was happening to me. To hide my blackouts, I would wait until the teacher and other students had left the room before getting up. I would even blackout and fall over when I got out of bed some mornings. I'd wait a few minutes before calmly getting up and getting myself ready for school.

It was a Friday when the psychiatrist, whom I now despised, gave me an ultimatum: eat over the weekend or go to hospital. It wasn't that black and white. I couldn't eat and he didn't understand why. Monday rolled around and I found myself sitting with my Mum in the emergency department of Monash Medical Centre. We sat there for hours and I refused food and water. We were eventually seen late in the evening by an emergency registrar who examined me. He told us there were no beds and that I would have to go home. He said I would have to get worse before I could be admitted. Mum was furious and I was ecstatic. I'd got my way.

As I was getting dressed to leave the cubicle, Mum started yelling at me. She screamed: 'Why are you doing this?' She was frustrated. She was watching me starve myself to death and it seemed as if no one wanted to, or could, help her. There was definitely no way she could talk any sense into me. Her anger at the hospital scared me. So, in a state of shock, I escaped from the cubicle, ran through emergency and sprinted across the hospital grounds until I was running down Clayton Road in the dark, almost drowning in the torrential rain.

I was about 400 metres from the hospital when I saw the headlights of a bus coming towards me. Soaking wet, short of breath and crying, I stopped and suddenly my sad little world dropped into slow motion. I remember thinking if I jump in front of that bus this torture will all be over. At that moment, on a miserable night in suburban Melbourne, I thought my life had spiralled out of control and I couldn't do anything about it.

Just as I contemplated jumping in front of the bus, a hospital security car skidded to a halt next to me and a guard grabbed me. I ended up back in the same hospital cubicle, right where I started. I was eventually sent home on the proviso that I see the adolescent paediatrician in charge at the hospital later that week. It was late when Mum and I finally headed home. It had been a long day.

I was admitted to the general Adolescent Unit at the Monash Medical Centre just two days after my close encounter with the bus. The paediatrician took one look and ordered me to go straight to hospital. Do not past go, do not collect $200. That was it. I wasn't even allowed to go home to get a change of clothes.

Wednesday, 24 August 1994

Here I am in Monash Hospital sitting in bed writing in my diary again. I hate this place already. I've been told I have anorexia nervosa but that's just rubbish. I know there's nothing wrong with me so why can't these doctors let me go home right now? I refuse to accept what they say about me. I'm angry with my family for putting me here. I'm angry with the doctors and nurses for keeping me here. I want to go home.

I'd never been away from my parents for more than a few days on a school camp, and even then I didn't like it. I didn't want to go to hospital. I was crying, 'Don't leave me here! I'm not staying here!' In hospital there was a pre-conceived idea that I was a little manipulative brat who had chosen this path in life. I could feel the judgmental attitude reflected in the eyes of the medical staff around me, burning my skin like a red-hot branding iron. I could already tell that I was viewed differently and more suspiciously than the other three patients sharing my room.

I didn't sleep at all that first night. There was continual noise around me; the high-pitched beep of a monitor in the shadowy distance, the soft murmurings of the nurses at their station just outside my room and the slow, heavy breathing of the boy in the bed next to me. I couldn't shut my brain off. I had thousands of thoughts racing around in my head. How did this happen, why was I lying in this hard and uncomfortable hospital bed?

Saturday, 27 August 1994

It's Saturday night and I'm lying in a hospital bed watching television. I wish I was at home with my family. I wish I could sleep. I've been trying really hard to eat today so that I don't have to have the tube on Monday but it's so difficult.

I was given the first weekend in hospital to show my doctor I would eat enough to avoid being fed by a naso-gastric tube. I really did try but everything was too much for me. On Monday morning I was given the dreaded enemy of an anorexic – the tube. My older brother Jordan was visiting me in hospital at the time and he had to walk away because it reduced him to tears to see me so distressed. He later told me he could hear me scream-ing from the other side of the hospital.

The first time they inserted the tube up my nose, down my throat and into my stomach was painful and humil-iating. A small length of the tube poked out of my nose and a bottle containing the liquid nutrition hung from a pole, much like an intravenous drip in hospital. The bottle was then attached to the end of the tube in my nose and would drip the liquid at a pace programmed by a small machine attached to the pole. I can still hear the sound of the machine as it pumped each drop into my tube, down into my stomach.

I was fed at night, the theory being I wouldn't be able to tamper with the feed if I was asleep. I couldn't tip the feed out and replace it with water, which happened most of the time during the day. This made no difference. I didn't sleep, so anytime was anorexia time.

The more hospital treatment I received, both psychiatric and medical, the more intertwined with my anorexia I became. Each admission to hospital saw me plummet to a new low. I began to learn and perfect the tricks of the eating disorder trade. I would barter with the dietician and doctors. I would agree to eat a certain amount of 'calories' if they would reduce the amount of feed I was given through my tube. I have never been much of a mathematician but when it came to food and calories I was as sharp as a calculator. The calories I agreed to eat would come in all forms, shapes and sizes. At times this posed a problem as my plan was to hide the food so I didn't have to eat at all.

Eventually, I agreed to eat the same amount in food as I was taking in by the tube. Having secured the deal, I would then hide all the real food and not eat a single thing. My anorexia was very clever. I would hide everything, including sandwiches, fruit and nuts, in my dirty washing to be sent home with Mum. I would water the plant or flowers beside my bed with my milk, orange juice and water. When there was no room left in my dirty clothes I would stash food in my clean clothes in the drawers in my room. This was very difficult to do as I had an observation window in my room and I could be seen from the nurses' station.

It all fell apart on Father's Day 1994 when Mum told the nurses I was hiding food. One of the nurses came into my room and declared she was going to perform a spot check of my belongings. It was like an embarrassing Customs check of luggage at an airport. She found nuts in my socks, bread in my T-shirt and a dead plant at my bedside. The list of hidden food was endless. As a result I was given a 'bolus', which is a large amount of Osmolite (liquid nutrition) inserted by syringe into my tube. I was mortified. My anorexia went crazy and I was extremely angry. They were not getting that stuff into me without a fight, I told myself, but in the end my family and the medical staff won.

Later that day I was weaving a cane basket as a gift for Dad. I had a pair of scissors and long strips of cane to make the basket. Still angry about the bolus, I grabbed the scissors and began hacking off my hair in big chunks. As soon as a nurse removed the offending weapon, I moved onto the next weapon. I made a jagged end on a piece of cane and began scraping it up and down the bare skin on my arms until they were red raw. I hated what I was and I thought I deserved to be punished. The same nurse rushed back in and confiscated everything around me except a blue Texta pen. Who would have thought a blue Texta could be a weapon? I sat there through the night painting every strand of my hair blue. It seemed I was always one step ahead of the nurses and doctors. Whenever they thought they had me cornered, I would find another way around them. Ideas would just jump into my mind without me even trying.

I was tube-fed for the next three weeks until I was discharged. I went home burning with determination to lose every kilo the hospital had made me put on. I started the second I got home.

Monday, 12 September 1994

I was discharged from hospital this morning. I packed my bags first thing in the morning but I had to wait until midday to see the doctor before being allowed to go home. Dad came and picked me up. My legs felt like jelly walking to the car because I'd been lying down for the past three weeks. I'm so happy to be home.

Thursday, 15 September 1994

I had to go back to Monash Hospital today to be weighed. I had to wait to see the doctor after a nurse weighed me. Apparently I've lost weight but I don't believe them or trust them. When the doctor turned up, she said if I lose any more weight I'll have to be re-admitted.

I knew how much I weighed at the start of every hospital admission and I would keep a track of it while I was in hospital. I was weighed twice a week and a chart was kept at the end of my bed, which was silly. Access to this sort of information was a wonderful thing for my negative mind and a dreadful thing for me.

My parents came to the conclusion that knowing my weight was not a good thing for me. It was clearly ammunition for my anorexia so they devised a plan with my doctors and the nurses to weigh me standing backwards so I couldn't see the numbers on the scale, and once recorded the chart was taken away. I was furious. At home, Mum threw out the bathroom scales so I had no means of finding out my weight, apart from going to the local shopping mall and weighing myself on a pair of scales for sale in Kmart.

When I wasn't in hospital, I still had to be weighed twice a week. One weigh day I was really anxious to know my weight so I called the hospital and pretended I was my Mum. 'Hi this is Jan Cullis,' I said. 'I would like to know what my daughter's weight was today.' The nurse, with no reason to doubt I was Jan Cullis, told me. I was an emotional wreck for the rest of the day.

It was around this time that I finally acknowledged I had a problem. I had been out of Ward 42 North, the general adolescent medical ward at Monash, for seven days and my health was going downhill fast. I had been trying really hard to eat but by the end of this particular week I just snapped. I tried over and over again to make myself purge. I cried with anger, but I couldn't let go of my feelings, until finally I went for a 3-hour jog. This was not normal for me. It was then that I knew something was terribly wrong.

Tuesday, 8 November 1994
A Letter to My Anorexia

Dear Anorexia,

Hi! Are you still lurking around up there? Isn't it about time you left? It's pointless you trying to rule me anymore! I'm too strong and I have too many people helping me beat you! You have successfully used all your tricks on me and it's my guess you have no more lurking up your sleeve.

I would like to tell you that I'm now aware of all your tricks and I know when you're trying to pull one on me. You might as well give up now because your tricks aren't going to work. You're not going to rule me anymore! You took my freedom from me. You took away my family and my life! You're a thief and I despise you. Why don't you just go and jump off a cliff? That's what you deserve. I want you to know that you're no friend of mine. You're not welcome anywhere near me.

*You had no right to intrude on my life the way you did.
I suppose I was a fool to listen to your dangerous
words that lead me down the path to disaster. This
was all your doing and I blame you for this.*

*I mean what I said earlier. Leave. There is no future
for you here.*

From your knowledgeable victim,
Bronte

It was common practice that after a few stints in hospital
with an eating disorder you would be shipped off to
the psychiatric ward, be it an adolescent or adult one.
After a few admissions, I was admitted to the Adolescent
Psychiatric Unit at Monash Medical Centre. My parents
and I were told that the unit would help treat my anorexia. My Mum and Dad wanted me to go. They were
desperate for anything to help. I, on the other hand, was
very sceptical.

The psychiatrists at Monash told me to write letters
to my anorexia thinking this would help me to identify
my illness. The truth is, the more letters I wrote to my
anorexia, the sicker I became. By November 1994, it had
been about eleven weeks since I was diagnosed with
anorexia. There seemed to be no easy solution. I was
getting worse.

Tuesday, 15 November 1994
A Letter To Myself

Dear Bronte,
*Well, I'm sitting here in these groovy hospital pyjamas
in Ward 42 North of Monash Medical Centre for the*

fifth time in three months. This time would have to be the worst though. No television, no telephone, no clothes – no anything! I'm isolated in a single room and let me tell you it's no fun in here. Well, it's not my cup of tea anyway. I have so many goals and hopefully by the time I read this letter back to myself I will have achieved some of those goals.

It's been one hell of a year! I think the hardest thing I could ever possibly do is try to beat my anorexia. I would never wish my negativity monster on anyone. 'He' is so strong and powerful. 'He' is also a bit of a trickster. I have to learn to tell 'him' to shove off because I need to eat. I may not want to but I need to eat if I'm going to stay out of the psychiatric ward.

I've spent the past five weeks in the Adolescent Psychiatric Unit. I really hate it and I don't think it has helped me all that much. I will get out of here on Friday and go back to the psych ward in the day and go home in the evenings.

I'm going to beat this damned ANOREXIA (otherwise commonly referred to as Negativity Monster). It has robbed me of so much: freedom, friends, independence, family and so on.

Luckily I know I can beat the hell out of it.

That I will do.

Love always,

Bronte

Wednesday, 16 November 1994

I know it sounds insane but I sometimes feel like there's someone inside me controlling my brain. I should never have let my weight, eating or what other people think *get the better of me, but unfortunately I'm not strong enough to fight. Life isn't always a bunch of roses!*

One thing I've learnt is that anorexia can happen to anyone. At first, you can control it until you get to a point where there's no control except for your will power to say NO. Being diagnosed with a disease of the mind known as anorexia nervosa was not an easy thing to accept. I seriously didn't think I had a problem. I realise things are wrong now, because as I write I'm sitting in hospital with a nasogastric tube stuck inside me feeding me liquid nutrients. If there was absolutely nothing wrong with me I suppose I wouldn't be here. Life is terribly confusing.

Thursday, 17 November 1994

How one can eat chips, chocolate cake, a milkshake and so on simply amazes me. I can't even drink a glass of water without feeling an overwhelming sense of guilt. I hate it. I want it to go away but it will not leave. Anorexia haunts me wherever I am, everyday of my life.

Bruises have started appearing on my legs. I bash my legs on things. I kick and hit myself. If I eat anything the pain gets worse and I have to harm myself even more to punish myself. It's the only way I can teach myself a lesson. Everyone learns from pain. Exercise is an essential daily activity but not for pleasure. My insides hurt and I feel worthless.

My intense need to burn off anything that went into my body through exercise was something my head turned into a ritual. At the age of fifteen, I began walking around the block obsessively. It got to the point where I had to do it a hundred times without stopping – and I had to do it everyday at the same time. One day Jordan just happened to be walking in the same street. He stopped to ask me what I was doing. When I couldn't answer him honestly, he grabbed me and physically stopped me from walking anymore. I panicked at being stopped because I thought something terrible would happen to a loved one. To protect my family I waited until Jordan left and I started my laps again – from the beginning.

Friday, 18 November 1994

I've learned to live without food – that's not the difficult part. The trouble started when I had to pretend I ate. Fiddling with the food didn't work so in the end I didn't hide it. I told them all I'm fat, I hate my body and I'm dieting.

My days seemed never-ending. They consisted of lying on the heater, riding, walking my dog, doing exercise and keeping up with school. I was under the care of so many doctors. There was my GP, psychologist, psychiatrist and a physician. The doctors told me that my muscles were wasting away and my organs would fail. I didn't believe them. It got to the point where the doctors would not let me go to school because I was in danger. I remember wanting to lose more weight and being happy when I lost 13 kilos in three weeks. I thought that was a good thing but no one else thought so. I couldn't understand why they weren't happy for me. I was so proud of myself.

I wasn't proud that I ended up in hospital. I was so angry about not having control over my life, my weight loss or gain. And I always felt like there was someone watching me, such as a doctor or my parents, every minute of the day. So much for my independence!

My weight was the one thing in my life I controlled but in a way I had no control. My weight loss spiralled way off track and I was pleased. I was so proud of myself but I didn't know that I was destroying everyone else around me in the process. Anorexia seemed like too much of a struggle to beat.

Saturday, 19 November 1994
My Monster

Trapped, motionlessly inside my own thoughts. Tricked into believing what is right and wrong. Surely this is not my ideal life, being ruled by a MONSTER more powerful than any other thought. The total power and control this monster creates is unknown to outsiders but not to me. It can't hide from me, nor can I from it. It hovers around day and night always present, whether visible or not. It's like being trapped in a cubicle made of glass. You can see life; see that it does exist. Friends, fun, excitement; it is all very visible and real but this MONSTER refuses to let me touch any of it.

I can see out of this glass cubicle but no one else can see in. Just me and my monster all alone and confiding in one another. I wish he would leave. I wait patiently for the day he gives up. Why did he choose me? Was I really that vulnerable and susceptible to his words? I argue constantly with him. I never give in without a fight. Sometimes I win when he is feeling weak. At other times he's much too strong for me to even argue with for I know he will often come out on top. But when I do win on those odd occasions, I feel like a little part of him dies. He becomes a little weaker but he is still there whispering things to me. He will leave, I'm positive he will. It will be one hell of a battle, but I'm just as strong as him and there is no way I'll let him win!

Along with sneaky behaviour came my many attempts to escape from hospital. I only ever succeeded once. On 1 December 1994, I ran away from the Adolescent Psychiatric Unit by removing the bars from the windows in my room with a screwdriver smuggled in by another patient. I somehow avoided the alarm system, slid under a hole in the wire fence and ran as fast as my legs would take me to the nearest train station.

Just as I was beginning life on the run, Dad arrived at the hospital to visit me. When he walked into my room to find an empty bed, an open window and curtains gently fluttering in the breeze, he shouted at the nurses, 'Where's my child?'

By that stage I'd bought a train ticket and I was standing on the platform when suddenly my psychiatrist turned up on the opposite platform. Thinking quickly, I left the train station and sprinted down the street. Like a scene from a film, I ran through a busy shopping area, side-stepping people and street stalls with a posse of hospital staff hot on my tail. I saw a bus and quickly jumped on board just as the doors closed behind me. I turned around and saw my pursuers in the middle of the street helplessly watching my government-supplied getaway vehicle trundle up the street. I was away.

I eventually got off the bus and hopped on a train into the city. I went to see my old friends at school. I don't know what I was trying to achieve. I wanted to run away from everyone and every thing but no matter how far I went, my anorexia was always there right inside me.

A teacher rang the hospital to say I was in the school grounds. Trying to keep one step ahead, I went to a friend's house and stayed there all afternoon. My friend made me drink some water as it had been one of those oppressively hot summer days in Melbourne.

I caught the train home that night thinking my parents would let me stay with them. I got home and I climbed over my neighbour's fence hoping to sneak in the house the back way so that no one would know I was there. The neighbour spotted me and rang my Dad. 'Bronte's just climbed over the fence,' he said. When I slipped inside the house I was greeted by an enraged father who dragged me to the car and drove me straight back to hospital. His anger that day is indescribable. I understand now that it came from a place of fear – a fear of me dying. I later found out that he, like the police and hospital staff, had been looking for me all day. It occurs to me now that running away in my condition was such a selfish thing to do to my family, but remember anorexia knows no logic. I couldn't see that back then.

The hospital put me in solitary confinement. I sat on a bed covered in white sheets, stared at white walls with no television, no radio, no clothes except a hospital gown, no books, no phone and no visitors for a month. I was told that for every meal I agreed to eat I would be allowed a privilege. I refused to eat and each day that passed saw me spiral further into my negative mind. These prehistoric tactics were actually fuelling my negative mind and reinforcing my ideas that I deserved nothing. Mum noticed that the treatment was making things worse and pleaded my case. Exasperated, the hospital gave up and let me have my things back. It was at this point that Mum began to understand that these professionals didn't have the answers and didn't understand my anorexia.

It was rare that there was only ever one eating disorder patient in the adolescent medical ward. There could be up to five at any one time but the average number was three. Another girl and I had both been in the same room for a few months when one of the younger nurses approached us and asked us how we lost weight so quickly. She wanted to know our secret, so to speak, so she could slim down and look beautiful. We offered to make her a meal plan. Two anorexics putting their internal calorie counters to work to come up with a foolproof plan for this very nice nurse. Imagine it!

I remember telling the many doctors that treated me that anorexia was not about weight. Yes, I was a concerned teenager and I had always thought and felt I was overweight, but this diet that turned into starvation was about so much more than losing weight. It was about the guilt that consumed me when I put anything in my mouth to the point that I wanted to die. I felt so worthless and unworthy of life that to nurture myself seemed wrong. I think that was why I was filled with guilt and anger when the doctors tried to save me. As time went on the need to control all the moments and events of my life became overwhelming. The voice and the inner thoughts that I thought would protect me from failing took over and wouldn't listen to reason. I watched as my life played out before me. I wanted to become invisible and eventually extinct. It was terribly difficult trying to explain these feelings to doctors and nurses when I couldn't fully comprehend them myself.

My negative mind was wearing a mask. The obsession with my weight, the number of kilograms, the obsession with looking in the mirror and thinking I was getting bigger with every glance – it was all a mask to hide my self loathing. It must have seemed to others that I was purposely manipulating everyone around me, but this was not the case. Again, my anorexia was very clever and deceptive. I was not. This was a very difficult thing for people around me to understand and so I would often go to bed in tears remembering the comments made about my so-called selfishness.

Wednesday, 7 December 1994

The psychiatrists here have told me to write a list of goals I want to achieve. Fair enough, so here they are:
MY GOALS
Short Term:
1. *Spend Christmas at home with my family.*
2. *Eat without hesitation.*
3. *Spend my 16th birthday at home.*
4. *Travel to Tasmania with my family.*
5. *Maintain my weight at 51–52 kg.*
6. *Go back to school part-time.*
7. *Stay out of hospital.*

8. *Spend time going out with friends.*
9. *Get back into life. Enjoy it.*

Long Term:
1. *Get back to school full time.*
2. *Travel overseas.*
3. *Get a part-time job.*
4. *Take up a physical hobby (such as netball or rollerblading).*
5. *Keep out of hospital.*
6. *Be healthy and fit.*

NB: *Read and look over these goals twice daily, until they are achieved.*

Wednesday, 8 December 1994
ANOREXIA
What has it taken away from me?
1. *My life*
2. *My family, home, brothers, sisters and two puppies*
3. *My school*
4. *My friends*
5. *My freedom*
6. *My happiness*
7. *Fun and excitement*
8. *Adventure*
9. *Physical activity*
10. *Outings*
11. *Opportunities*

What has it given to me?
1. *Misery*
2. *Restrictions*
3. *Unhappiness*
4. *Negativity*
5. *No freedom*
6. *A life spent in hospital*
7. *Disputes and anger with my family*
8. *Knowledge of who I am*
9. *A lot of anger*

NB: *Read over these twice a day. Once in the morning and once in the afternoon for as long as I think I will need to.*

A WEB OF DESTRUCTION

Lost in his power, never to be found. Too strong for me, too strong to Argue with, too strong to bother with, much too strong to beat. Now, I dont even notice he's there. If Im following his commands, he blends in, I dont notice him, but if Im trying to be myself then he comes down on me hard. I began my battle alongside him. Then I fought him on my own. Slowly an Army emerged behind me, trying to help, but I denied them. Now the army has dissapeared and he and I have once again joined forces, fighting against everyone and everything. Fighting against freedom and hapiness. No long being able to differenciate him from me. He is a part of me or should I say I am a miniscule part of him. I am my own enemy. I can no longer sense when he is tricking me. I sometimes wonder if it really is him or if it's just me conjuring things up in my wild Imagination. Maybe he contrd my imagination aswell. It's as if everyday he is spreading inch by inch infesting and slowly taking over my whole body. My dream is to Run away and be a carefree spirit. Run away from Him, even if it's only for one day. Run away, do and be what I want, not feel bad, guilty, angry, depressed, nothing. Feel nothing feelings hurt too much. No direction, nothing. A WORLD FULL OF NOTHING BUT PAIN CAUSED BY HIM. CAUGHT IN HIS WEB OF DESTRUCTION WITH NO WAY OUT.

1995

Thursday, 23 March 1995
School English Essay

As a teenager of the world today I have many dreams and goals. I also have high expectations of myself. I want so much to finish school and continue on with further education in the arts, graphics or journalism. I also want to help others in the world. However, I have been somewhat setback due to an illness that imposes on and rules my life. About a year ago I was diagnosed with an illness common among girls of my age, anorexia nervosa. I've spent the past 7 months in hospital receiving both medical and psychiatric treatment. The battle is not over yet and I still have a long way to travel but with my family's help I have hope that, with time, I will beat this monster that has taken my life away from me.

Friday, 21 April 1995

It's almost 5 p.m. and I have a really big decision to make. I can either drink heaps of orange juice and eat an apple or I can have a nasogastric tube inserted into my nose. What would you do? I definitely don't want the tube but there's no way I can drink four cups of orange juice all at once. I could have a go at tipping the

juice down the sink but I really haven't had an oppor-
tunity yet with all these nurses around me. I've already
thrown away heaps of food and that makes me feel
a lot better. I just can't believe I'm back in hospital
again. I'm so angry at life.

A nurse was doing her observation rounds one night when she came to me and whispered in my ear, 'You don't deserve the bed you are lying in. You're a manipulative little bitch and someone who is truly sick deserves this bed. You deserve to die.' Everyone except my family seemed to think that I was behaving and thinking like this on purpose. It made me ask myself if I was creating all of this with my wild imagination. Despite that, there was a part of me that knew I couldn't help what was happening. I couldn't stop it. It was out of control and I would wonder how anyone could possibly think I could deliberately torture myself. Most people I encountered in the hospital treated me as a lesser human being who didn't deserve treatment. I wasn't really sick, they said, like people suffering from cancer, renal failure or diabetes. All that the treatment in the hospital, both physically and psychologically, taught me was that everything I believed about myself was true. I was less deserving. I wasn't worth helping.

Wednesday, 31 May 1995

Tonight I got a big SCARE. It really was a horrible experi-
ence. Something told me to throw away half my
cheese. I'm not sure why I even did it. Anyway, the nurse
found it in the bin and said I had to have another bolus.
A bolus is 350 calories in liquid form pumped into my

nasogastric tube compared to the 30 calories that I threw away. So anyway, I refused the bolus. She said I had to have it and that's all there is to it. I still refused so she rang the doctor who also said I had to have the bolus. I then cut a deal. I said I would eat all the cheese if they didn't give me the bolus, which is exactly what I did. So I narrowly escaped the dreaded bolus but I spent an hour crying my eyes out. I have a major headache now and I feel really depressed.

I have to get weighed tomorrow and I'm really frightened. I'm not asking about my weight any more. It makes me too angry. The doctors put my medication for obsessive-compulsive disorder up to 25mg of anti-depressants a day, which is one tablet. I hope it doesn't make me sick like it used to. I almost died because of low blood pressure the first time I took one of these tablets and I ended up in emergency.

I hope the tablets work because it would be great to get out of the big black hole which I have got myself stuck in. It would also be great to get rid of the voices and thoughts and worries that go round and round in my head. Over and over and over!

Dad finishes work in two weeks. I feel really bad about him quitting to care for me at home. I have myself to blame for everything that happens. Everything seems to be my fault. I just want to get out there and get on with life. I've been trying really hard to eat my meal plan, so that's one step forward. I'm only eating my meals because I don't want the bolus but at least that makes me eat. Something has to. That's all for now.

Monday, 12 June 1995

I'm really sick of being in hospital. I keep putting on so much weight. I hate putting on weight. I feel so incredibly fat in here. Life is so unfair sometimes. I've been in hospital for eight weeks straight.

Living with anorexia was a daily struggle not only for me but also for my family. As my Mum once remarked, 'Bronte doesn't have anorexia, our whole family has anorexia.' My parents suffered, my siblings suffered and my grandparents suffered. Anyone who loved me suffered in his or her own way.

We didn't know a thing about eating disorders when I was first diagnosed with anorexia. It was extremely difficult for my family, and myself for that matter, to understand why I was behaving this way. They, like most of the world, thought I wasn't eating by choice. They were so frustrated with me, especially my older brother Jordan. One Sunday night in 1995, Jordan videotaped the movie, *The Karen Carpenter Story*, hoping I could see what I was doing to myself. Karen died of a cardiac arrest caused by the strain anorexia put on her heart. She was thirty-two. Jordan wanted to give the tape to me in hospital but it never arrived. Angry and confused, he smashed the tape against a wall at home. This was the beginning of the end of our friendship. Anorexia destroyed the good relationships in my life, starting with my family.

In July 1995 my parents signed me out of hospital to care for me at home. I was to be tube-fed and, in order to keep me safe, it was decided that Dad would quit work to be my carer – to keep me alive. Mum continued working to bring in a wage to keep the rest of the family alive. Dad spent every minute of the day with me until Mum got home from work at 6 p.m. when they would do a changing of the guard, so to speak. Dad would take off to his escape, coaching and refereeing basketball at night.

It might seem that Mum got the easier part of the deal as she only had me for a shorter period in the evening. This wasn't really the case. Dad spent more time with me, and he had to deal with more meals and weigh days, but Mum got the job of monitoring the nasogastric feed every night and often I would sleep in her bed. This was not an easy job as anorexia and I were tricky customers.

On more than a few occasions Mum would come into the bedroom late at night to find that I had cut the end of my tube, disconnecting it from my liquid food supply. I thought this would mean no feed that night but all it meant was a trip to the hospital at some ungodly hour to have the tube painfully replaced back up my nose. Other nights, Mum would wake up to find her bed soaking wet and sticky. I would make a nick in the tube in the hope that the mattress rather than my body would absorb most of my feed. It was a never-ending battle. I was a 24-hour-a-day job.

Sunday, 2 July 1995

Well, it's been about a month since I've written in my diary and I'm rather ashamed of myself. This month is the first anniversary of my ANOREXIA. I know it's nothing to be proud of but it's a fact.

Anyway I'm pretty tired so I might go to sleep now. Goodnight. I'll tell you more later on.

Friday, 7 July 1995

Well, nothing really exciting has happened. Oh yeah, except I was in the paper and on TV and I've been out of hospital for two weeks – a record-breaking time for me. About this TV thing, I was on the Today Show on Channel Nine, which was very scary and embarrassing. Mum, Dad and I were on television for an interview with Liz Hayes about anorexia and how to care for a sufferer at home. It went for about five minutes and, let me tell you, it was not a nice experience. I never want to be on television again!

Mum and I were also in The Australian newspaper for the same reason. It seems other people are fascinated by my anorexia. It was all very new and exciting but at the same time it was extremely scary.

I never wanted to be on television. I never wanted my face on television. My family didn't want to be on television. I didn't want my 15 minutes of fame. But I got it.

People often ask me how the television cameras ever found me. After all, I was just a very sick teenage girl dying in suburban Melbourne. Whenever people ask me how I ended up on television, my answer never changes – I'm not really sure. I don't remember a defining moment when I agreed to have my torment and despair splashed on Australian and New Zealand television. I don't remember my parents saying, 'Hey, Bronte, can Channel Nine come over and film you while you're dying?' To be honest, I really don't know how it became what it did. I don't have strong memories of the start of the whole media frenzy. So much of it is a blur due to the depth of my illness.

I appeared on the *Today Show* and in *The Australian* in July 1995 but it wasn't until Neil Mitchell interviewed me on Radio 3AW in Melbourne that it all took off. That was after I had been discharged from hospital to be cared for by Mum and Dad at home. There was an issue. Now that I was being cared for at home instead of hospital, my parents had to pay for the very expensive nutritional supplement needed to keep me alive. Previously it had been supplied as part of the hospital system but now my parents had to pay for it, which seemed ludicrous. My Mum had to say something publicly about it and somehow we ended up talking to Neil. As it turned out, he didn't just ask about the high cost of care, he wanted to know about my anorexia, or as Mum would say, our family's anorexia.

As we were talking away in the radio studio, Margie Bashfield, a producer from *A Current Affair* on Channel Nine, was listening and almost crashed her car as she listened to my Mum describe the madness we were all going through. Margie went straight to the office and told everyone about this amazing story she had heard on the radio and pretty quickly tracked Mum down. My reluctant television saga was about to begin.

Sunday, 16 July 1995

I was just looking through my diary from last year and I found a poem I wrote about my anorexia. I will copy it down in here:

> *There she sits, huddled in the corner,*
> *No escape or way out.*
> *At first it was in her control, but now it controls her.*

The nightmare lives on and doesn't ever disappear,
It's there, night and day lurking around the next
corner.
It is so strong and overpowering;
To beat it or even fight it is impossible.
But one day it will die and when it does, she will be
free once more.

Thursday, 20 July 1995

Today was quite a challenge. Actually, the past few weeks have been a struggle for me but I've survived. I've stayed out of hospital for four weeks now which is such a good record for me. I think I've probably spent a total of a month at home in the past year. I've been admitted to the psychiatric ward at Monash Hospital twice and it really didn't do all that much for me. Dad is now at home helping me to get better. I can't believe he did something like that for me. I appreciate and love him so much. I wish there was something I could do to thank him. We are really poor now because of me. I feel bad about it because Dad left work for me.

I'm still getting the nasogastric tube at night. I got weighed today and I really didn't enjoy it. I lost only 100 grams.

Thursday, 28 September 1995

About a week ago I got so fed up with it all that I did something really stupid. I took an overdose of 35 anti-depressant tablets. I had to go to the hospital and get the drugs out of my body. I was in hospital for a few days as the drugs I took were very dangerous. I was so

scared that I was going to die. I have such an impor-
tant and exciting life ahead of me. There is so much I
want and need to do with my life.

I didn't want to die but in a way I considered myself to
be dead already. I don't know if I can fully explain the
torture I was suffering or the intensity of my anorexia
and its control over me. I was tired and resigned to the
fact that I would never recover. My doctors were telling
my family and me that I was going to die and that we just
had to wait until it happened. I'd lost all hope and I had
no more faith left in living.

As I sit here writing I'm fighting back the tears
because this is something I like to pretend never happened. I've never really talked about my overdose. I
remember the events of the day so clearly. I had returned
home from hospital and I was on one of those 'I'm
going to get myself better' kicks. But no matter how
hard I tried to get myself better, nothing seemed to
change.

It was a spring day in Melbourne. Late September
back in '95. I was sitting huddled over a heating air vent
at home. I was freezing – I always seemed to be cold no
matter the weather when I was sick – and I had so many
anorexia-driven thoughts running through my head.
Everything I did was driven by anorexia. It had infil-
trated my whole being. There was no way I could separate
anorexia from me, or me from anorexia.

Usually when I was overwhelmed by negative
thoughts I would bang my head on the ground to make
them stop, but this day was different. Dad wasn't home;
he was out coaching his basketball team. Mum and my

younger brother James had been in Canada for a week checking out the Montreux Clinic. Jordan and Sam were around somewhere but I was alone and I felt like no one else existed except my anorexia. I wanted to escape and rest for a minute, to not think about anything. I wanted everything to stop. My doctor had prescribed an anti-depressant pill a day to help me cope with my obsessive-compulsive behaviour. But this day I had an entire packet of anti-depressants in my grasp and in a moment of desperation, I took every single pill washed down with several glasses of water. The moment I swallowed the last one, I panicked and ran to Jordan and confessed. He promptly screamed at me and told me that if I ever did anything like that again he would never speak to me.

Jordan drove me to my local GP and then I was taken by ambulance to Monash Medical Centre. I remember lying in the emergency ward in silence with two tubes up my nose, one forcing liquid charcoal into my stomach, another supplying nutrients to keep my heart pumping and an intravenous drip in my arm. I hated myself even more for how selfish I'd been by not thinking about what I was doing to my family. It was a night that never seemed to end where each minute seemed like a lifetime. Dad sat beside my bed the entire time. I wonder how each minute felt for him. I wonder what it must have been like for him to call Mum in Canada and tell her the news. And what about Mum, half a world away from her youngest daughter who had just overdosed?

The next day I saw a doctor from the psychiatric department who asked me why I had attempted suicide. My answer was that I hadn't tried to kill myself. All I wanted was an escape from the hell I was going through. In taking the overdose, it gave me ammunition to hate myself even more for being what I considered a weak and useless person who couldn't stop the desire to escape from a hard life.

I now understand that I wasn't weak but I was extremely sick and in a place where no other solution seemed to exist. I was actually strong enough to ask Jordan for help when I realised the overdose was going to cause pain, not make it go away. Even today it still baffles me that I could see clearly how an overdose would hurt my family, yet couldn't see the hurt I was causing my family by starving myself to death. That's anorexia for you.

Saturday, 30 September 1995

At the moment I'm in the car on my way to Sydney. Dad is driving and Nanna is with us. We are staying in Sydney for a week with my Nanna's sister, my great aunty Thel who's just had a heart operation.

So much has happened since I last wrote in this diary. Firstly, I've been back in hospital. Things were going really well at home until I started tipping out my nasogastric feed. I then began losing weight really quickly. I stayed in hospital for two-and-a-half weeks and my weight didn't really change from when I first went in. I was 46.4 kg when I went in and when I left I was 47.4 kg. So much happened when I was in there. I kept tipping out my feed so the nurses started taping the tube up and watching me like a hawk. I chucked a few wobblies while I was in there. I cut my hair again, tried to run away twice and cried every day. Hospital is just not my kind of place.

**

Our lives were being destroyed by anorexia, I was dying and my family was falling apart, both mentally and physically. Dad said they felt swamped by anorexia because they, like most Australians, didn't know what this strange disease was all about. Sam and Jordan hate anorexia, which is understandable when you consider what it did to them and what it stole from them. Jordan tried so hard to convince me to eat. When he failed, he became angry and avoided coming home in case he saw me. More than once he said my anorexia took his parents away. Almost overnight, the attention of two parents was focused on just one child. Sam, Jordan and James became orphans. In hindsight, my parents admit that concentrating just on me was a mistake.

James was the worst affected. Just weeks before leaving for Canada, Mum and Dad found James crying as he rode his bike in circles in the dark. He couldn't come inside the house because of my anorexia but he couldn't escape it outside either. He was trapped within the family's invisible walls of pain. Even though she was frustrated with my anorexia, Sam would defend me to the hilt. In her final year of medicine she walked out on a lecturer discussing eating disorders. She was upset and disgusted at having been told that her sister was manipulative, her father a molester and her family dysfunctional.

I still feel incredibly guilty about the impact my illness had on my brothers and sister. The worst part is that nothing will ever give us back the childhood or youth we should have had together.

Monday, 2 October 1995

Well, we've made it to Sydney after our long drive.
Despite being tired we're all looking forward to explor-
ing Sydney.

Mum and James aren't with us because they're still
in Canada looking at an eating disorder clinic for me.
I just know the lady who runs the clinic won't want
to know about me. But I appreciate Mum and James
going halfway around the world to get help for me.
I'm so sick of living with this stupid anorexia. It's
ruining our lives. I feel so guilty all the time. I hate it.

I'm missing Mum terribly and, surprisingly, I miss
James as well.

Mum stood banging on the solid timber front door of an
old house, hoping someone would answer. As she waited
for a sign of life, Mum took a moment to look over her
shoulder at the quiet suburban neighbourhood. Cherry
blossom trees lined the street. This was the other side of
the world, Canada, and she was in a pretty town called
Victoria that hosted the 1994 Commonwealth Games.
But this wasn't a holiday. Twenty hours earlier Mum and
James had set out on a mission to save my life. Now here
she was in a strange country, growing more impatient by
the moment. Mum knocked again and again. 'Come on,'
she whispered. She knew she'd taken a gamble by coming all this way without an appointment but she knew
she had no choice. She was about to knock again when
suddenly the door opened.

Mum has always been close to her younger brother
Bryan. He married Mum's lifelong friend Bronte; that's

how I got my name. They live in Utah in the United States. Uncle Bryan and Aunty Bronte were watching television one Sunday evening in 1994 when they saw an episode of the *20/20* current affairs program about the unorthodox Montreux Clinic saving the lives of eating disorder sufferers. They called Mum and told her about the clinic. Excited by this glimmer of hope, Mum faxed the clinic.

After five months of trying to get a response from Montreux, Mum, Uncle Bryan and Aunty Bronte decided they couldn't wait any longer. My health had deteriorated to the point where the doctors said I was going to die. Mum met with Uncle Bryan and Aunty Bronte in Canada and they all found themselves, along with James, standing on Montreux's porch, at 1560 Rockland Avenue, banging on the front door.

Mum was relieved when a man called Noah finally greeted them. He told them Montreux didn't receive unannounced visitors. Mum explained she'd travelled all the way from Australia but Noah said people from all over the world were landing on their doorstep every day. You need an appointment, he repeated. Mum begged him to ask if anyone had heard of Bronte Cullis as she had been faxing and phoning for five months. He closed the door to check leaving Mum, Uncle Bryan, Aunty Bronte and James standing on the porch for what seemed like an eternity. Just as they were about to give up, Noah returned. They had been granted an audience with Peggy Claude-Pierre.

Peggy Claude-Pierre was a softly spoken Canadian who always seemed to care about you. She was a good listener. Her defined features, pale complexion and blonde frizzy hair sat in contrast to her black Armani jeans and her black Armani jacket. In fact, Peggy always seemed to wear the same black clothes. She must have had a wardrobe full of the same outfits! All the staff appeared to wear black and they all drove black cars. Black was certainly the Montreux colour of choice.

Peggy told the Cullis party she would help me and gave them an admission date for eight months' time. Until then, she said, they had to keep me alive. Mum, Uncle Bryan, Aunty Bronte and James walked down quiet, conservative Rockland Avenue back to their city hotel crying but not speaking. The sun was shining and it was a beautiful day.

The next day, my team got up early for the walk from their hotel back to Montreux to sort out the paperwork. Grey clouds and rain had replaced the sunshine. When they arrived, they were let in straightaway this time, and taken to the office where they got the biggest shock of all. The cost of treatment at Montreux was US$30,000 per month. They were speechless until Uncle Bryan chimed in with, 'Not a problem, we can do that.'

Monday, 30 October 1995

I don't like Mondays. I've been horrible and mean to absolutely everyone today. I feel really awful about it but I can't help getting angry. I was weighed today. It was terrible as I'd put on 400 grams. I just can't handle gaining any weight. One gram is way too much for me. They want me to maintain my weight but I don't even want to do that. I have my mind set on losing weight. Sometimes I wish I could weigh nothing. I weigh 44.5 kg and I can't handle it. I want to be less so badly. I want to be 37 kg and maybe then I might be happy.

Tuesday, 31 October 1995

Mum and James have just returned from their trip to the US and Canada. James had a wonderful time, especially with our cousins in Utah. Mum had a good time at the clinic in Victoria, Canada. She learned a lot from Peggy – the lady who runs the clinic – and returned home with a changed attitude and so much more understanding of anorexia. Mum told me about the workers and explained that most are 'lay' people while some are recovered anorexics and or bulimics who had been through the Montreux program. She told me of the love that exists at Montreux and promised me that it was different to Monash and the treatment I've received so far.

Wednesday, 1 November 1995

This morning Mum and Dad went on Radio 3AW again to talk about anorexia and the Montreux Clinic in Canada. Mum also spoke about the terrible way sufferers are treated by some hospitals. It upset me a little bit but hopefully it will help raise awareness of anorexia and maybe we could get a clinic here. It could also help raise funds as Mum says Montreux is very expensive. I feel so bad about all the money people are paying for me. I feel so guilty.

About seven months before I left for Canada, the tone and attitude of the Monash Hospital staff changed. It's truly amazing how when one person opens their mind, others are more inclined to follow. The nurse in charge at the Adolescent Unit at Monash had known me since my first admission and initially she'd been very hostile toward me. She had the same pre-conceived ideas as everyone else.

The penny finally dropped for her when, at Mum's suggestion, she watched the tape of the *20/20* television show that had given us hope. She then showed it to her team. From that point on she became loving towards me and became my protector from others living in ignorance. When my fear of calories jumping on me intensified, she would pick me up and rock me in a chair until I was calm. She let Mum sleep next to my hospital bed and she let my family stay with me 24 hours a day to protect me from my negative mind. Compassion entered the ward and was passed onto other sufferers.

Wednesday, 8 November 1995

Ray Martin is coming to our house tonight to meet us and talk to us. I've had the camera crew with me for the past few weeks but I haven't had to say anything to them. I feel scared and nervous when they're around. I'm really quite terrified of Ray coming.

I wasn't home when Ray arrived. I vaguely remember disappearing on purpose because Mum had told me Ray and his television crew were coming to our home. Anyway, Mum tracked me down and said, 'Ray's here, you better come home.'

My first meeting with Ray Martin was very difficult because unlike the camera crew who just watched, he was full of questions that I didn't know how to, or want to, answer. It was terribly hard to speak to someone I didn't know or trust about my torment and torture.

I was suffering and didn't fully understand it myself at the time so how on Earth could I explain it to someone else, especially someone famous with a camera recording everything I did and said?

The first story about me, my family and our anorexia ended up as two stories. At the end of the first night's filming, the camera crew packed up their gear and drove off. The discussion was about what they had just witnessed and recorded. This story – my story – wasn't like your run-of-the-mill current affairs fodder, they concluded. The story of the Cullis family madness and anorexia deserved wider coverage.

The camera crew lived at our house day and night for several weeks and followed us to hospital, out shopping, anywhere. My family wanted to show the world what anorexia was really like.

I didn't like watching myself on television – in my condition, who would? In fact, I have hardly ever watched myself. It's too painful and the times I did watch, I ended up in tears. So why did I agree to appear on television a few more times? Quite simply it was the thought that maybe I could help other sufferers. Perhaps one parent could learn something and change their child. At the time, I didn't think anorexia had ever been portrayed the way it really was for me. All I really wanted to do was help people see that my anorexia wasn't just about food.

My family and I received hundreds of letters from viewers who watched that first story on *A Current Affair* on 20 November 1995. Many people gave money to help me get to Canada. Most letters were from average

Australians who wanted to give a little something to help another person. They gave never knowing if I would ever come home alive.

Wednesday, 22 November 1995

I'm in hiding as I write this. The Channel Nine cameras and a big television truck are here but this time Mum and Dad will be talking live to Ray Martin in a studio in Sydney. Apparently Canadian Airlines saw the story the other night and have decided to give Mum and me a free ticket to Montreux. Why are these people helping me? I mean, it's nice, but why waste the money on me?

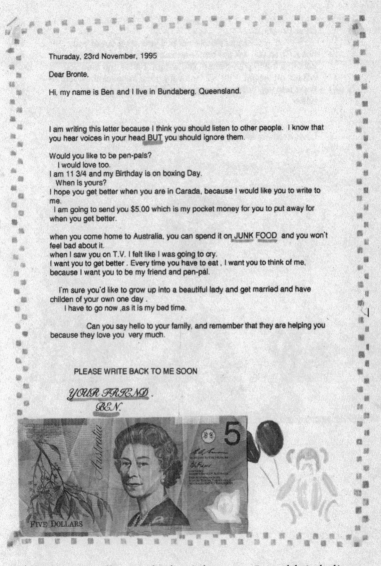

Thursday, 23rd November, 1995

Dear Bronte,

Hi, my name is Ben and I live in Bundaberg, Queensland.

I am writing this letter because I think you should listen to other people. I know that you hear voices in your head BUT you should ignore them.

Would you like to be pen-pals?
I would love too.
I am 11 3/4 and my Birthday is on boxing Day.
When is yours?
I hope you get better when you are in Canada, because I would like you to write to me.
I am going to send you $5.00 which is my pocket money for you to put away for when you get better.

when you come home to Australia, you can spend it on JUNK FOOD and you won't feel bad about it.
when I saw you on T.V. I felt like I was going to cry.
I want you to get better . Every time you have to eat , I want you to think of me, because I want you to be my friend and pen-pal.

I'm sure you'd like to grow up into a beautiful lady and get married and have childen of your own one day .
I have to go now ,as it is my bed time.

Can you say hello to your family, and remember that they are helping you because they love you very much.

PLEASE WRITE BACK TO ME SOON

YOUR FRIEND .
BEN.

Ben's letter really touched me because I couldn't believe a boy would send me $5 of his pocket money to help me get better in Canada. I still have that same $5 note.

Dear Bronte,
        Can you please not pull your tube out of your
nose. Then you will get better and eat your breakfast and
your lunch and your dinner. You will get better and then you
will put on weight. You will look very good in the clothes you
wear and you will look very pretty because you will get
better.

Love from Kristin (6)

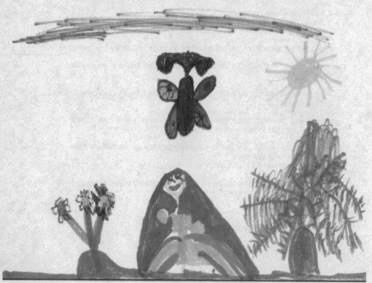

Dear Bronte ,

   My name is Briony and a think that you are wasting away to a
twig. If you think you are fat that must make Elle MacPherson obese , many people
will agree that you need a big feeding , you need some fattening if you ever want to
grow up and get married , you'll have to eat food , anyway your family will always
love you no matter if you are fat or skinny and nobody should judge you on your looks
or how you dress because it's your personality that makes you who you are not what
you look like.

    From Briony (12 years old)

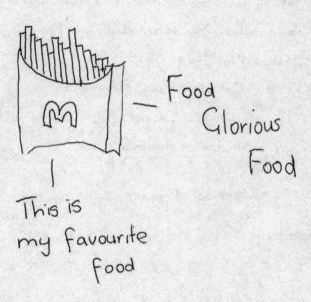

— Food
Glorious
Food

This is
my favourite
food

Hi Bronty
            My name is Jessica.
I'm eleven years old. On T.V. I saw the pictures
of when you were younger. I thought you
were beautiful. And I hope you start eating
and get better. Don't hurt your self Bronty.
We all get cross but that is no reason hurt
our selves. Your parents Love you Bronty
they wouldn't lie to you.

            Get better soon Bronty.
    If you ever feel like writing to me my address
    is at the top of the page.

    Thinking of you

                                Love Jess ♥

Dear Bronte'

This card is for all the
Christmasses you have to look
forward too,

Fight the voices , Bronte, they
can be beatten . Wage World war 3
on them and never, never give
up. I know, I've heard them
too.

You will win in the end.

Good Luck , although you
do not need it.

Jenny T.

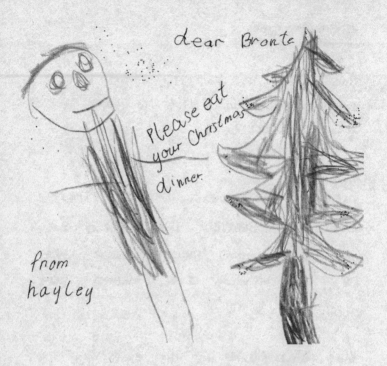

dear Bronte

Please eat
your Christmas
dinner.

from
hayley

1996

Wednesday, 3 January 1996

It's my 17th birthday today and guess who I celebrated it with? My wonderful family – of course – and Channel Nine! They want to do another story about my last birthday before I go to Canada. That's if we find enough money to make it over there. I find it so hard to pretend to enjoy myself when I despise who I am. All I really want to do is stay in my room. I don't know why anyone wants to make a fuss over me.

Anyway, I decided to bake a cake for my birthday. I made sure I had gloves on while I was making it so the calories couldn't jump onto my hands. I didn't eat any cake but everyone else seemed to enjoy it.

I was convinced that calories could jump. I believed that all I had to do to ingest food was to look at it. I thought that if I was around food then the calories would jump on me and get under my skin. I spent most of the time holed up in my bedroom with towels rolled up to plug the gaps under the doors to stop the calories getting in. When I wasn't in my room, I would pull my jumper over my head to walk around the house just in case someone was eating. I would do the same thing to get past the kitchen regardless if someone was eating there or not. I couldn't even be around people who had just eaten; somehow I thought they would make me fat. As Dad looked after me during the day, I had to follow him everywhere including grocery shopping at the local supermarket at Rowville. I hated grocery shopping days. As you can imagine, with all these thoughts I had, the supermarket was a very evil place. Every time I went I was convinced the calories would accost me in the aisles and that I would leave looking like the size of a blimp. After every shopping trip I would go home and shower to scrub away all the supermarket calories and the germs from just being in public.

While Dad was at home looking after me he started his own diary. Looking back at parts of it, I can get an idea of what he went through. His reality and my reality were so far apart.

Dad's Diary

Thursday, 8 February 1996

I had to wake Bronte today as she had an appointment with the psychiatrist at 9.30 a.m. Of course, she wouldn't eat or drink this morning as it was also a weigh day. After the appointment, Bronte seemed quite OK. She said the doctor had discussed what would happen at the Montreux Clinic and that it was different from the Adolescent Psychiatric Unit at the Monash Medical Centre. Bronte seemed happy with his explanation although I don't really know how he knows what happens at the clinic.

In Ward 42 South there were only four patients so the

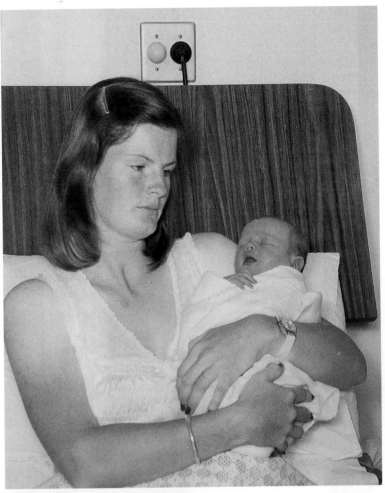

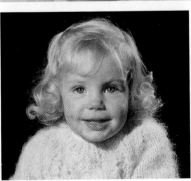

Above: My Mum and me at the hospital the day I was born, 3 January 1979.
Left: Me, age two.

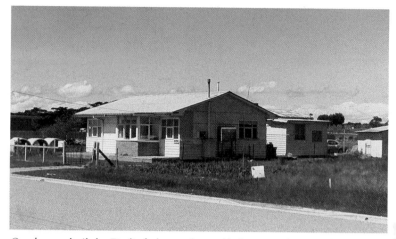

Our house, built by Dad's father and grandfather, at Safety Beach on the Mornington Peninsula in Victoria.

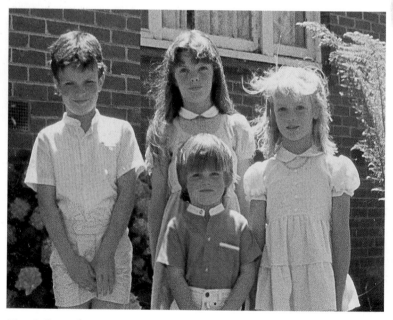

The Cullis Kids in the front yard of our house in Garfield in the Gippsland District, Victoria, during the summer of 1984. Jordan and Sam are in the back row and James and I are in the front.

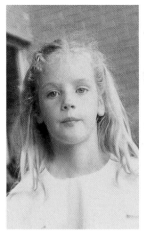

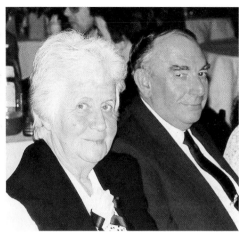

Me, age eight.

Nanna and Poppa Cullis.

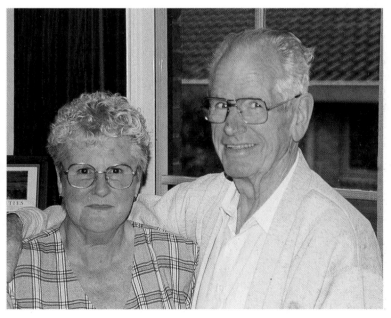

Nanny and Poppa Clarke.

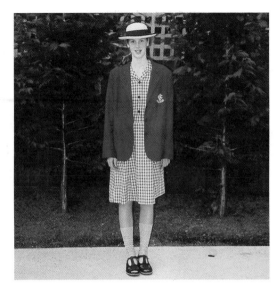

Me, age 14, in the backyard of our house at Rowville.

Calories - Monday 28th/11/94.

Breakfast - 16.

(140 + 115) = 255.
Lunch - 70×2 + 85 + 30

Dinner - 30 + 70 + 73 + 60.
       143. 283.
SUPPER - 200 + 65 + 70 = 335.

(65
 + 70   255
 135   + 283
            + 335
            + 16
            839 calories

839 calories
+ 20.
859
= 859 calories for the day!

Anorexia doing the maths.

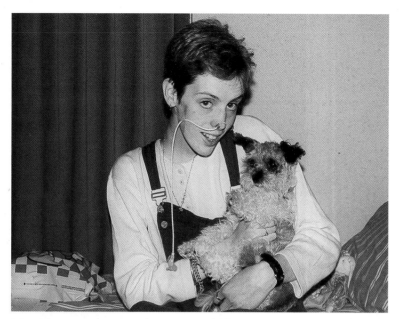

Me with my nasogastric tube in 1995, cuddling our little dog Muffin.

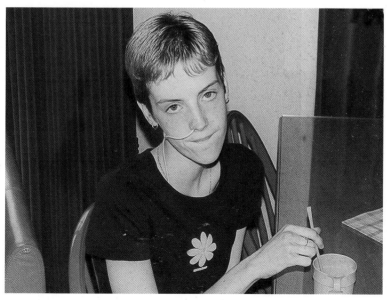

Me trying to avoid taking a sip of water and unhappy about the camera being there.

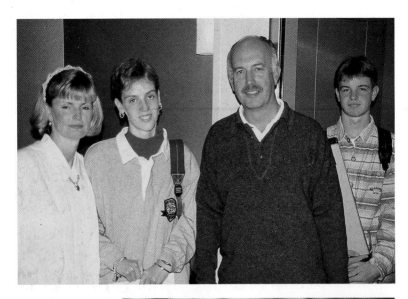

Mum, me, Dad and James at Melbourne airport before boarding the plane for Canada on 28 April 1996.

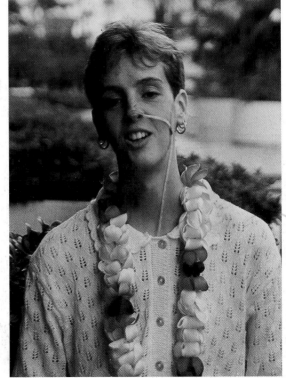

Me wearing the lei I made during our stopover in Hawaii on the way to Canada.

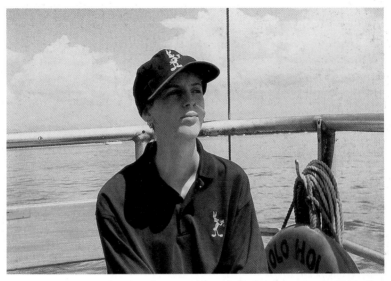

Sitting at the back of a glass-bottomed boat on a family outing in Hawaii.

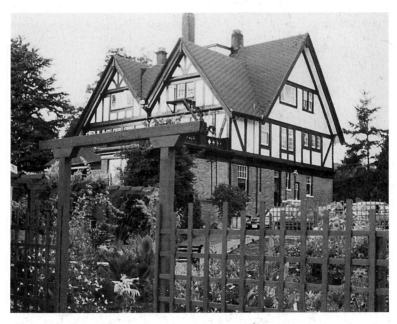

St Charles House at the Montreux Clinic.

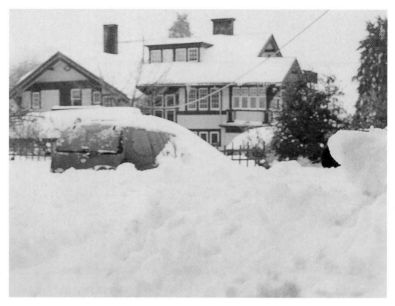

A view of the back of the Mansion during the snowstorm of 1996.

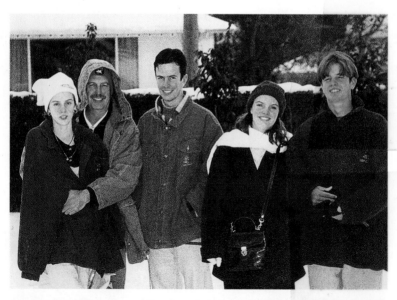

Me, Dad, Jordan, Sam and James gathered on the Mansion's snow-covered front lawn for a family photo during their surprise visit at Christmas 1996.

nurses didn't have much to do. One of the nurses took Bronte into a room to do the weighing and observation. I went in with Bronte to ensure that she didn't see her weight, which stressed her out. I also didn't see the weight.

During the weighing process it was obvious by the nurse's face that she did not like or approve of Bronte's behaviour. While Bronte was getting dressed I went to the nurse to find out Bronte's weight. She said it was 44.4 kg. I was surprised because I would have thought she had lost weight.

She offered to re-weigh her but it was too late. Bronte was out of there. I chased her down the stairs, which seems to be the norm now, and I tried to cheer her up by assuring her that she was not fat and generally trying to make light of the situation. It didn't work as usual and I was punched a few times, scowled at and told how much I was hated. That also seems to be the norm these days.

When I got to the car, I got in and started the engine but Bronte kept walking. I quickly got out and chased after her. After a struggle to get her in the car I was walking around to get in when she locked all the doors. It was cold, windy and wet and I didn't have a jumper. I was freezing. I sat on a fence under a tree watching her scream, cry, hit her head and scribble all over her arm with a pen.

After about 15 minutes she jumped out of the car and ran across the oval nearby. I grabbed the keys, chased her down and brought her back to the car. We went to my parents to visit as we had arranged. I should have known better as she made the visit uncomfortable and we had to leave. At home I had to watch her all day and, of course, she refused all food and drink because she thought she had put on weight.

Bronte was almost uncontrollable this afternoon so I went to Jan's school. Sometimes that helps her to calm down but *this time it didn't. I became angry and frustrated so I left her there and went home. Next thing I know Pat, my mother-in-law, arrives. Jan couldn't handle Bronte so she called in a reinforcement. I went to train my Under 10 basketball team then referee all night. When I got home I discovered Bronte had been admitted to hospital yet again. It turns out she tried the pretend she was Jan routine again and convinced a nurse to tell her weight. All hell broke loose according to all reports including my neighbour. Jan rang the hospital and told them that Bronte had ripped out the nasal tube, cut her hair and was now uncontrollable. The hospital sedated her, inserted a new tube and fed her osmolite. I slept in my bed and it was heaven.*

Observation: *Bronte's resourcefulness and inability to think logically is incredible.*

Friday, 9 February 1996

Bronte rang this morning to say she was allowed home and that she was ready to be picked up. I'd enjoyed the night without the responsibility of Bronte and I was not in a hurry to go to the hospital. When I arrived Bronte was ready and packed. She was apologetic.

Observation: *Always seems subdued when being discharged from hospital. Also wants to do everything possible.*

Saturday, 10 February 1996

I cleaned up around the house before getting Bronte up and feeding her breakfast: two Weet-Bix, 100 ml milk and 200 ml of orange juice. Jan was still in bed so I went and got in with her. We were lying there for a moment when Bronte came into the room. She began to get angry and after some discussion it turned out she didn't want us in bed.

She wanted us to get up. I conned her into bed with us and gave her a cuddle and she was all right.

For lunch I fed Bronte one piece of wholemeal bread, one slice of cheese and 200 ml of orange juice. I took her to the house of another anorexic, Olivia. They went to the pictures but she came home early because she couldn't cope with the clutter at Olivia's house.

Observation: Jealousy. Can't cope with idleness. Can't handle clutter or untidiness.

Sunday, 11 February 1996

Bronte was bored today so Jan and I offered her a number of activities or chores to do but she refused. She quickly worked herself into a state and announced that she was leaving home and not coming back. I had to run after her and drag her back. After a while she calmed down and we worked on the computer together.

I took some time off this afternoon while Jan took Bronte to the movies. As usual, the outing was a testing time for Jan and Bronte.

It was difficult to get Bronte to go to bed tonight so finally I went with her. Jan had to do some schoolwork all night.

Observation: It seems that Bronte requires our attention all her waking moments.

Mum had the job of caring for me on weekends so she'd try to find things to occupy my mind. One thing I loved to do was going to the movies. When I first became really sick, a movie outing was a great distraction from all the things going on inside my crazy head. But, there's always a but, it wasn't such a great outing for Mum.

As the demons in my mind were taking over I started to believe that I could somehow absorb calories out of thin air. Imagine what it was like going to the movies and walking past the candy bar? And have you ever looked under the seats of a busy cinema? No need for me to do that. I knew there was popcorn and other bits of discarded food lurking under the seats and hiding up the aisles ready to pounce and smother me with calories. Mum would always go in first, like a president's advance security party, to clear a path free of food. My one-woman SWAT team would get down on all fours to crawl along our aisle picking up popcorn and clearing the seats of any stray food wrappers. That done, Mum would then block access to the aisle until this eagle had finally landed safely.

Dad's Diary

Thursday, 15 February 1996

TODAY IS WEIGH DAY! Bronte wouldn't have a shower so I picked her up and started carrying her to the car. She quickly promised that she would have her shower so I took her back inside but she didn't keep her promise so I carried her back to the car without a shower. That certainly set the pattern for the rest of the day.

At the hospital, the charge nurse weighed Bronte. She said she didn't need me to go in with Bronte because she could handle her. It wasn't long before I heard the wailing from the room and words to the effect: 'I saw!' When Bronte came out the nurse spoke to her for some time to try to keep her calm. It didn't work. Bronte had worked herself into a state so we had to leave.

On the way out Bronte was screaming and wailing and all eyes were on us. Even at this early stage I was threatening to take Bronte back up to Ward 42 South. The people around us must have thought we were crazy. I was losing it even at this early stage. I finally grabbed her wrist and dragged her screaming all the way to the car. She yelled: 'I hate you, I'll run away, I won't eat again, I put on over a kilo, I saw my weight. I weigh 44.2 kilos'.

I don't understand why she did it but she threw a few punches, which hurt. I had to force her into the car and the self-abuse started. Hair pulling, kicking herself, etc. When we got home Bronte went for scissors, knives and even blunt instruments to hurt herself. I had to follow her, hug her, hold her and try to convince her that what she was doing was not the best thing. Fortunately I was able to talk her out of pulling her tube out. I had to threaten her but hey, it worked.

Everyone was trying very hard to be nice to Bronte but she distorted everything that was said and done for her. Pat [Bronte's grandmother], seemed to cop a barrage of abuse and hatred. I felt very sorry for her.

Of course, Bronte wouldn't eat or drink and there was no point in trying to make her.

Observation: *A little worse than a typical weigh day. Something must change.*

Weigh days were horrific for everyone. There were occasions, quite a few actually, where I wanted to just kick or smash the television camera into pieces and tell the crew to get away from me. I was in so much pain sometimes that I didn't want anyone to see me suffering. The days I was weighed at Monash were extremely hard for me to handle. Sometimes the camera crew waited outside, with our blessing, for my reaction after I'd been weighed. One day I really lost it in front of the camera. I had just been weighed and I was distraught because I sensed I had put on weight (I didn't know at the time because the nurse would never tell me the weight but I could just feel it) and I certainly didn't want a television camera watching me. I sat in the gutter crying and shouting at Dad who calmly kept telling me how much he loved me. The more he said he loved me, the angrier I got and the more I shouted back, 'I hate you!' Eventually, he picked me up and put me in the car. He thought that was that but then I locked all the doors. I felt like a monkey in the zoo with people watching, pointing and saying, 'Hey, look at that freak!'

Another weigh day turned really ugly. As I was running out of the hospital, I was confronted by a cameraman waiting at the door. I was as angry as hell and I just wanted to smash his camera to pieces and shout, 'Get lost!' I don't know why I didn't. I guess something told me that holding the camera and microphone were innocent people who would also become victims of my anorexia. I held back my feeling of destroying the camera crew and all that came with it. Cameraman Mick Morris, sound recordist Joe Ferma and producer Margie Bashfield eventually became my friends.

Dad's Diary

Friday, 16 February 1996

I had to referee some basketball games tonight so I left Bronte with Jan. Before I got away there was a heated debate as

Bronte negotiated a new meal plan. I chickened out and left them to it. Because of Bronte's attitude, Jan rang Monash Hospital and spoke to the charge nurse. She arranged for a doctor to call back. Later that night a doctor rang and advised Jan that Bronte would have to be admitted through casualty for treatment. Jan put up a strong argument against this. Nothing was resolved over the phone.

We need to speak to Bronte's paediatrician to help develop a contingency plan for the future. Bronte took the osmolite tonight only because she knew she was dehydrating and we reduced the amount from one litre to 800 ml.

Observation: *The hospital does not seem to want to help or cooperate with us.*

Saturday, 17 February 1996

Bronte appeared much happier today probably because she finally got her own way with the meal plan. I feel weak to give in but I also feel relieved she's calmed down. I've told her that if she requires hospitalisation it will be on her head. Of course that was a waste of breath as she forgets everything and she cannot follow logic.

While I was out Jan rang the Montreux Clinic to get some information sent out to be part of her submission for funding for a curriculum about eating disorders. Bronte got to speak to the accountant Celine about the clinic which appeared to have a soothing affect on her.

Today Bronte ate her lunch and her dinner and had water and 400 ml of orange juice.

Observation: *Things are heading in the right direction again.*

Wednesday, 21 February 1996

Bronte accepted all her food and drink today. I think it was because she will be weighed tomorrow. She went to the movies to see 'Sabrina' with her grandmother and her cousins.

I went to visit my old work mates at Croydon today. I spent most of my time talking about anorexia and Bronte because she was on TV.

Observation: *Sometimes this anorexia gets too much.*

Thursday, 22 February 1996

Bronte went to Monash Medical Centre for her weekly weigh-in. I knew she'd lost weight but the nurses wouldn't tell me how much. It's a new policy because of Bronte's condition. The doctors were not available so we left. At first Bronte appeared reasonable but out of the blue she got angry, hit me, dug her fingernails into my arm and refused to co-operate. When she got angry I told her that she'd lost weight and that deep down she knew that also. At first she said she hadn't lost weight, then she said it was probably only 100 g. I asked her why she was so angry and she replied that I would make her put on weight. We had the usual show of yelling and screaming as we left the hospital. It seems that I'm still hated on Thursdays.

Bronte refused to eat all day and had very little fluid. I gave her a full can (946 ml) of osmolite that night. Well what a performance, she wouldn't go to sleep and Jan could not handle it so that night I made Bronte sleep in her bed and I slept in Samantha's bed. I think I got about two hours sleep the whole night.

Observation: *Put on weight or lose weight Bronte gets angry.*

Friday, 23 February 1996

Bronte refused to have her breakfast but ate her other meals. She never seems to get tired. Another late night, I'm bushed.

Observation: *Bronte never seems to be tired.*

Sunday, 25 February 1996

I've just fed Bronte her breakfast. Oops, I forgot her drink so I'll give it to her now. I bet she carries on because I remembered.

Back now and I was wrong. She laughed and then sighed. Hang on, no I wasn't wrong. She's now angry and wants to tip it out. My life is bliss! Got to go for now.

Back again! Jan bought a deckchair this afternoon for Bronte. When she got home Bronte sat on the deck writing and reading. She finally looked content. Ah, but pretty soon she was angry again, screaming and throwing things around the house. Apparently she didn't say her prayers long enough and they weren't said in the right order. I made her come outside and stain the decking with me. That helped a lot!

Later that evening I found Bronte in her room praying. The prayer went on for about 30 minutes until I made her stop. Soon after I found her doing exercises in her room. She waited up until I organised her osmolite for the night and then she went to bed. I don't think she had enough fluids today.

Observation: *She must be kept occupied.*

Bronte's Diary

Sunday, 25 February 1996

It's pretty warm, about 30 degrees, and I'm sitting out on a deckchair Mum bought me. I've got so many things going through my head, so many thoughts

*about life. The voice in my head is pretty strong and
very scary. I hate the way it threatens me. It's not very
fair that I have to live with these horrible thoughts and
the guilt feelings and the hatred of food. I wish I could
just be normal like everyone else. I wish I could be
happy.*

*We have been pretty busy lately. Yesterday, we had
a garage sale to raise money for me to go to the clinic
in Canada. We raised around about $1500 which was
pretty good for a garage sale. I'm getting pretty hot
sitting out here. I'll write more later.*

Dad's Diary

Tuesday, 27 February 1996

*Bronte would not eat breakfast today. We were all bored
because of the rain which limits her activities. For something
to do, we went to the shops to buy food for a roast dinner.*

*We then came home and watched television this after-
noon. Bronte cracked it again for some reason, but we're used
to it. She thought she had a valid reason but I couldn't understand what the reason was. I had to stop her hurting her head
on the floor. Her voice is strong at the moment and causing
her hell. She is praying and exercising obsessively.*

Observation: *She is heading for another stint in hospital.*

Dad was on the couch watching television one afternoon
trying to take a break from the relentless grind of caring
for me. I was sitting quietly on the cool tiled floor not far
from him but my eyes weren't on the TV. I was staring at
the floor, pre-occupied with a battle raging within me.

The voice in my head was screeching at me creating a cacophony that was unbearable. No matter what I did I couldn't stop the voice telling me I was worthless. I couldn't make the voice shut up so I leant forward and sharply bashed my head on the tiles as hard as I could. I did it again and again hoping the voices would stop. Within an instant, Dad had leaped on my back and restrained me in a wrestler's headlock. Apparently, he asked me what the hell I was doing. At the time, I couldn't answer him. All I could hear was the negative voice I couldn't silence.

People often ask me about the voice, or thoughts, in my head. Well, the day I bashed my head on the floor is an example of what it was like before I left for Canada. Back then the voice wouldn't leave me alone and I often whacked my head in a crazy attempt to make the voice go away. I felt like I was drowning in appalling thoughts about myself. It was like I was a hostage and my kidnapper, anorexia, had a gun to my head shouting, 'I will kill you!'

Dad's Diary

Wednesday, 28 February 1996

It's difficult to get Bronte to eat all the food on her meal plan. I'm past fighting her. As far as I am concerned, roll on 28 April when we take Bronte to Canada. I haven't given up on Bronte — I'm just very tired.

Bronte's voice is giving her hell. Her obsessions are currently:

* *Praying. She has to say the same thing over and over again and they go on forever.*
* *Washing hands after she touches anything.*

· Exercising a set number of times in a particular way.

She knows these obsessions are weird. She often cries during the day and tells me that she can't live with the voice anymore and if she doesn't get better she doesn't want to live. The voices tell her that if she doesn't exercise or pray or wash her hands or whatever, she'll get AIDS (another paranoia) or she'll get fatter or she'll not go to Canada.

Jasmina, a neighbour, asked Bronte if she would like to watch her kids play tennis. I told Bronte to go. About 15 minutes later I received a phone call from Bronte who was crying and blubbering about someone who was eating food at the court. I had to pick her up. I feel like I'm a slave to her emotions.

I fed Bronte when I got home and there was a lot of screaming. I had to go to bed with her until she went to sleep because her mother had lots of schoolwork to complete especially after today's incident with Jan's hand. I really love Bronte but it is hard right now.

Observation: *I'm her emotional crutch.*

One afternoon in early 1996, Mum walked home after a day teaching at the local primary school. Before she could even see the house she could hear the screams from the battlefield that was the Cullis family home. She didn't have house keys so she knocked on the front door to be let in but no one could hear her over the shouting. Suddenly a rage erupted from deep inside. Angry and frustrated, she punched her fist through a glass panel in the front door, cutting her hand. Ignored and defeated, Mum turned around and walked to the doctor to get the wound stitched up. Such was the depth of her emotions back then. She was in the trenches fighting anorexia in ugly hand-to-hand combat and she didn't want to lose the war. Losing the war meant losing her daughter.

Dad's Diary

Thursday, 29 February 1996

It's Thursday so it must be weigh day. I found out her weight from last week. She had lost nearly 2 kilos in a week. Today, she weighed exactly the same as the week before. I was able to talk to Bronte's paediatrician for a while and I told her what Bronte was up to and that I'd reduced her feed and why I'd reduced it. It was agreed that she would talk to Jan and me a bit later about how we would handle Bronte as we get closer to leaving for Canada. She also suggested that Bronte should stay in hospital the week before we leave. That way the medical report could be written up in the best environment.

As Bronte and I were leaving the hospital it was as though she had to react so the abuse started and she got angry. It was nowhere as bad as other visits. Of course, she wouldn't eat or drink all day.

We went home and I went to basketball training for the last time. I then went off to referee some games. This time is my release as I leave Bronte with Jan. When I got home at 11.30 p.m., Bronte was still up and wanted to know if she could change her pyjamas because she thought that there were calories on them and that she'd get fat. I said NO and sent her to bed.

Observation: *Better than most weigh days but her phobias are getting worse.*

Friday, 1 March 1996

*Bronte's compulsive behaviours — exercise, prayer and hand
washing — are getting to the ridiculous stage and I often won't
let her do them. I don't know if it's the right thing to do but
I know letting her do them doesn't help. In my view, it makes
her worse. When I stop her, she yells and screams that she has
to do them all over again, right from the beginning.*

Observation: *We need help to stop her compulsive
behaviour.*

My germ phobia got out of control and continued to get
worse as time went on. I started to wash my hands more
often until it got to the point where I had to wash them
after everything I touched. As a result my hands were
cracked, bleeding and extremely sore, although I wouldn't
admit it at the time. There were days when I just wanted
to distract myself and try to get lost in something else.
I tried to use television as a distraction but I soon started
thinking that if I didn't get up and wash my hands at every
commercial break that not only would I become a huge fat
pig but something would happen to Mum or Dad.

As my illness grew stronger and I grew weaker, the
irrational thoughts became more powerful and more real
to me. I can see how ridiculously untrue they are today
and I wonder how I could have possibly believed those
things. At the time they were very real.

Dad's Diary

Saturday, 2 March 1996

*My Under 10 basketball team won today! They were on the
bottom of the ladder and we beat the top team. To celebrate,*

we all went to McDonald's. Discussion inevitably turned to Bronte and anorexia. It's amazing how many people have come into contact with anorexia. I know they mean well — and it's an opportunity to explain to the best of my knowledge what anorexia is about — but sometimes I wish it would all go away.

I fed Bronte when I got home tonight. I don't know why she won't eat for Jan. I can get her to eat even if she objects, most times anyway.

It was announced that there was a change in Government and that John Howard is the Prime Minister.

Observation: *Bronte is jealous of her time with me and Jan. She is like a little girl.*

Bronte's Diary

Sunday, 3 March 1996

I've had a pretty awful day because my voice has been at me all the time driving me crazy. I had a big fight with Mum over lunch and I feel guilty for starting it.

The past week was terrible. I spent a lot of it crying or worrying about something. I'm so sick of living like this. I got weighed on Thursday and Dad said my weight stayed the same. I don't know whether to believe him or not. I can't stand getting weighed. It makes me so mad. I was mad all Thursday so we cut breakfast out of my meal plan but now Dad wants to add it back in. I don't know what to do. I'll feel so bad and guilty if I have breakfast again. I wish I were normal.

It's 56 days until we leave for the clinic in Canada. It's two months away and seems like forever. I wish I were there now.

Dad's Diary

Sunday, 3 March 1996

I just washed out Bronte's nasogastric tube. She was asleep but she woke as soon as I touched the tube. She did her usual complaining and half cry but it was flushed anyway. When I left she shut her eyes.

Observation: *It's amazing how lightly Bronte sleeps.*

Tuesday, 12 March 1996

Today was hell. The voice in Bronte's head is so strong. I've been trying to get her to eat three times a day. So far I've been unsuccessful. I made some breakfast for her consisting of one Weet-Bix and 50 ml of milk. She refused to eat it. She was abusive and angry and regrettably I lost control when she clamped her mouth shut. I threw the food in her face, turned the bowl upside down on her head and poured the orange juice over the top. I really regretted doing it for two reasons. Firstly, because I felt sorry for Bronte because I knew it wouldn't help her and secondly because I had to clean up the mess.

Later, Bronte and I talked about the problem and we both apologised for our behaviour.

Bronte and I went out to collect Jan's birthday cake.

Observation: *Bronte is stubborn.*

Tuesday, 12 March 1996 was a bad day. Dad lost the plot trying to feed me breakfast. He must have felt as if he were hitting his head against a brick wall as he hand fed me like a baby day after day. Dad can't exactly remember what started it this day. He thinks it was the grinding, relentless and repetitive nature of fighting anorexia that got to him. Dad was always reassuring me, trying to allay my fears about food, at this time. It was always the same dialogue from Dad, 'There's no extra milk in it, there's no fat in it, there's no this in it, there's no that in it'. One day Dad cracked. He picked up the bowl of Weet-Bix, tipped it upside down on my head and then put it down very calmly. There was no yelling. Then he picked up the orange juice and started to pour it over my head. He was halfway through with the orange juice when he realised he'd made a hell of a mess in the kitchen. He picked me up, clothes and all, walked into the bathroom, sat me in the shower, turned the water on and went back to clean up the kitchen.

Mind you, I didn't go without my breakfast that day. After the shower we started from the beginning with Dad measuring out the food while I questioned and argued. Dad now knows that by tipping food over me, all he was doing was strengthening my anorexia.

Dad's Diary

Thursday, 14 March 1996

Weigh day. I got Bronte up and we went to the hospital for the weekly weighing. She didn't seem to be overly disturbed today. We had a few whimpers on the way out but nothing substantial. She didn't eat until dinnertime. I left Bronte with Jan while I went to basketball. Bronte went to sleep very late.

Observation: *Strangely subdued. Something's around the corner.*

Friday, 15 March 1996

I finally got Bronte out of bed at 11 a.m. and by the time she showered and got dressed it was the afternoon. I fed her lunch and then we watched a movie together.

Bronte's obsessive behaviour is out of control. I had to keep her with me all afternoon because of her obsessive praying, exercising, showering and washing her face.

James and I refereed a basketball game tonight. When Jan picked me up I discovered that Bronte had collapsed and was taken to the GP for treatment. The hospital doesn't appear to help us much even though we have taken over her care. These days if Bronte needs hospitalisation we have to go through the emergency system — and that takes hours. After careful consideration we decided to care for her at home until Monday but we put the hospital on notice that if anything should happen to Bronte we would hold them responsible. Bronte was fainting and she actually asked for a drink of water.

Observation: *We need to sort out the hospital.*

Saturday, 16 March 1996

It's Jan's birthday. Jan took Bronte to the doctor to have her blood pressure and heart rate checked (OBS, as the doctor calls it). While they were gone, I prepared a party breakfast for Jan. When they got back Jan's parents were here visiting for her birthday.

Bronte was very unstable and was on bedrest. Fortunately Jan's sister Gail looked after her while we went out. I've noticed that when Bronte is this unstable she doesn't put up much resistance. We all stayed home that night and watched a movie.

Observation: *When she is really unstable there is little if any resistance.*

Monday, 18 March 1996

Jan took the day off work and we both went to the hospital to have Bronte checked out and to see the paediatrician. Bronte was at her lowest weight of 41.4 kg and her OBS were unsatisfactory and so she was admitted immediately. The plan for her was extra food and fluids, which she found very difficult. I spent the day with Bronte convincing her that she must eat and I was successful. I got home about 9.30 p.m. and went to bed.

Wednesday, 19 March until Sunday, 31 March 1996

I went to the hospital every day to feed Bronte her meals. Usually I would go in early in the morning for her breakfast and stay for lunch and then go home about 1.30 p.m. I'd then return about 6 p.m. for dinner.

It appears as if Jan doesn't want to go to the hospital at all. When she does, she doesn't stay long and leaves immediately the meal is over. This was obvious to Bronte and it concerned her.

In many respects it's easier with Bronte in hospital but in other ways it's harder to juggle the time required with Bronte and time required with the other children.

Monday, 1 April 1996

Jan's brother Bryan, his wife Bronte and their six children have arrived from the US. They wanted to see Bronte before heading off to Adelaide so I hitched a lift with them to the hospital. We were running late so I rang to ask the charge nurse to please feed Bronte before we got there. When we arrived Bronte was still eating breakfast and struggling because we could hear the howling as we approached the ward. Bryan and Bronte and the kids waited for a while and I suggested that they head off as I wasn't sure how long Bronte would be. I think the howling made them a bit uncomfortable so they left with some reservation.

I waited for the paediatrician in the hallway with Bronte. I wanted to keep an eye on her as she had tried to run away. The paediatrician agreed that Bronte could come home provided she stays on the same meal plan. The grin on Bronte's face went from ear to ear. It was good to see her smile. She then tried to negotiate a lesser meal plan but it was made clear there was no negotiating otherwise she'd have to stay. She reluctantly agreed. I knew then that I'd have trouble at home with the meal plan.

Thursday, 4 April 1996

Jan took the day off work as we had things to organise with the travel agent. While she did that, I took Bronte to be weighed at the hospital. She wouldn't eat breakfast, of course, before the weighing. It was pretty much the usual weigh-in story. The stressing out, the claims that she's put on weight saying that she saw the scales and that she is a fat pig, yelling and physically hurting herself. It becomes very tiresome. With the charge nurse's help we were able to feed Bronte her breakfast. Her OBS were stable, which was the main thing, but her weight had remained the same. It's been as difficult as I suspected to keep her on that meal plan at home plus her activity rate has increased since Bryan, Bronte and the kids have been here. She remained in her bad mood for the rest of the day. Jan and I ate a snack at the shopping centre and Bronte sat away from us because we had food.

Friday, 5 April 1996

I escaped early this morning and spent the day refereeing at a basketball tournament. I left Bronte to Jan for the whole day. It was a welcome relief for me. I had to give Bronte her dinner which is usually more difficult after Jan has fed her during the day but we got through it.

Part Three

Montreux Clinic

Saturday, 27 April 1996

We're leaving for Canada in the morning. Mum, Dad and James are coming with me. I'm feeling so nervous and scared about going to the clinic but I'm also relieved that I'm going.

There's a party going on at home tonight to send me off but I refuse to leave the bedroom. I'll just sit here and try to watch television. I'm consumed by all these negative thoughts about my future.

I never liked watching American talk show host David Letterman until one very sleepless April night in 1996. His show seemed so much more interesting this night because it was the only thing on television that could partially take my mind off the thousands of thoughts, and the nerves, consuming me about the day ahead. My emotions were torn. I wanted that night to never end, like the dream where you're running along a road that goes on forever. But I was also anxious to get the next day over and done with. The arrival of this next day had been my reason to live for the past seven months. The longest seven months of my life.

The day before we left was one of chaotic organisation. Have we packed this, have we packed that, what about our visas, the airline tickets . . . where are the tickets? The drill of preparing and the stress before flying was intense because my parents were travelling with a terribly sick child. Not only did we have to take luggage for four people, we also had to pack enough Osmolite to keep me alive during the five-day journey to Canada.

A farewell party was thrown for me the night before we left. Of course, with food being served at the party I, the guest of honour, didn't attend. Instead, I sat huddled on the floor of Mum and Dad's bedroom, which had become my bedroom during my illness.

There I was sitting on the floor of my adopted space trying to protect myself from everything bad on the other side of the door. There were two doors into this room, one through the ensuite bathroom and the other was the entrance to the hallway. I was terrified of an imaginary army of calories creeping under the doors and infesting my body with fat, a bit like a scene from a B-grade horror film. A party down the hall and two doors to guard made my job of keeping the calories at bay a lot harder. I grabbed every towel I could find and shoved them under and around the doors to fill all the gaps that could potentially let the calories slip in to attack me.

My extended family were at the party and so were a few close family friends. A Channel Nine camera crew was also at our house to record the whole leaving event for the television saga. I could hear noises of 'life' happening around me, which magnified my feeling of utter self-loathing. I was so useless, I told myself, that I didn't deserve that 'life' I could hear. The conversations I couldn't hear at the time were centred on whether I would survive the Hawaii stopover and make it to Canada alive, and whether anyone would ever see me again.

I only let one person into my guarded space that night and that was Scott, Samantha's boyfriend. I don't know why I let him in. Scott was always very good at making me laugh and perhaps I felt bad that he had been exposed to our family madness. Our conversation was short but very powerful and I treasure it to this day. He told me that I didn't need to worry about Sam because he would always look after her. This eased some of my fears of leaving my family and reminded me that they had each other. As he left, Scott gave me a hardcover black book to write and draw how I felt when I couldn't express myself. I wrote to my diary like I was writing to a trusted friend. I felt safe doing this as I knew my diary couldn't be judgemental, it couldn't talk back, it would always listen. It was the one thing I felt I could be honest with and it's where my truths were kept. I still have it with me.

At 3 a.m. it was time to load up the car with our luggage for the trip to the airport. I was in tears as we stepped out into the cold night air terrified of what lay ahead, afraid of the unknown. It was a pitch-black night and there must have been some clouds slowly drifting overhead, as I couldn't see the moon. I stood in the driveway crying and clutching our dog, Muffin, begging to take her with me to Canada. Dad prised Muffin away from me and I got into the car.

Melbourne's Tullamarine airport was quite crowded for four in the morning. There was another family farewell committee waiting for me, which I found quite overwhelming because I didn't know some of the people. As Mum, Dad, James and I boarded the plane for our six o'clock departure, the realisation hit me that I didn't know if I would see the rest of my family again.

The Channel Nine camera crew filmed as we boarded the plane. They had organised a window seat for me and I clearly remember the sound recordist, Joe Ferma, waving goodbye from the air bridge. I waved back as the camera recorded and then suddenly the plane was taxiing towards the runway. Joe, cameraman Mick Morris and producer Margie Bashfield all wondered if they would ever see me again. Joe said it was a horrible feeling standing there waving goodbye. He hoped and prayed that the clinic in Canada would help but the truth was he just didn't know.

The fact that I was actually leaving everyone I loved hadn't sunk in until the Canadian Airlines 747 was sitting on the runway ready for take-off. Before this moment, the voice in my head had me convinced I wasn't really going. But I was. It was 6 a.m. on 28 April 1996. Later that day Martin Bryant would murder thirty-five people in Tasmania in what became known as The Port Arthur Massacre.

My doctors allowed me to fly to Canada on one condition, that I rested along the way to stabilise my health. They thought being locked in planes for almost a day, the time it took to get to Montreux, and locked away from emergency help could kill me. This meant three days in Hawaii, which turned out to be a nightmare for us. I was extremely phobic by this stage and I couldn't really cope with life.

Many things happened in Hawaii that sent me into the deep end with my anorexia. As we checked in to our hotel in Honolulu, I remember seeing some brochures promoting lei making courses in the lobby. I thought that might be a bit of fun and a distraction after such a long and painful flight. What started out as a good idea, gently threading metal skewers through the flowers, quickly descended into chaos when I pricked my hand with a skewer. I started screaming, 'I've got AIDS, I've got AIDS.' Quick as a flash, Mum called Dad over, grabbed his hand and stabbed him with a skewer. She asked Dad if he thought he had AIDS? 'No,' he replied, 'but that bloody well hurt.'

Our next attempt at quality family time in Hawaii was a trip in a glass bottom boat. The ticket seller assured us that there would be no food on board. 'It's not allowed,' he said as he pointed to a sign. We sat at the back of the boat with everyone staring at me. At least it seemed like that at the time. My emaciated body, nasogastric tube and cropped hair made me look like I had a terminal illness. A well-meaning man wandered over and sat beside Mum while chomping on a bag of potato chips. He was asking Mum what was wrong with me when I saw the food. I tried to throw myself overboard but Dad moved quickly and wrestled me to the ground. Mum also leapt into action yelling, 'Everyone with food, go to the front of the boat quickly!'

We left Hawaii for a 5-hour Canadian Airlines flight to Vancouver followed by a 45-minute flight to the tiny airport on Vancouver Island. I was feeling totally exhausted by the time we landed as were Mum, Dad and James. As I stepped onto the tarmac I saw two guys, one holding a television camera and the other a microphone pole, and the only thing I could think was, 'Are these guys ever going to go away?'

We had a day and a half to kill until I was officially admitted to the Montreux Clinic. The time dragged on, seconds felt like minutes and minutes felt like hours. It was spring in Canada when we arrived which meant rain and cold weather. I later learnt that the spring of 1996 was actually quite mild but it certainly didn't seem like it to us. To keep the time moving, and James and I busy, Mum and Dad decided to take us whale watching. The wind was ferocious that day and it was sleeting. I had never been so cold in all my life and I actually felt frozen to the core. I was battered and bruised the next day from the rough ride and in retrospect we probably should have done something a little less risky and something my body could stand up to but at the time it wasn't the natural elements that bothered me. It was the fact that I was so dead inside that I didn't even recognise the natural beauty around me.

I clearly remember every detail of the hotel room where I spent the last night with my family before entering Montreux. The walls were painted hospital white and the heavy smell of an oil heater lingered in the air. Marble tiles lined the bathroom floor, which supported an old-fashioned claw foot bath. I remember some unusually large seagulls perched on the windowsill hanging around in the hope of food scraps. Boy, did those birds pick the wrong room that night. I don't know why my memory of this room is so strong when many other events of that time are a blur.

On my first day at Montreux, a carer, Louise, was waiting for me in my new home, a two-bedroom apartment called the Pink Suite. I didn't speak to Louise, or anyone else, that afternoon. She could only watch as I broke into bout after bout of tears. The afternoon merged into the evening. Darkness swept through the room as Louise was replaced by another carer. I lay on the bed with my face buried in a pillow. I don't remember exchanging a word with my evening carer, although I remember exactly what she said to me. 'You will not leave until you are well.' Oh great, I thought. I'll never leave this place. I was already a prisoner of anorexia and now I was a prisoner of these strange people in this strange place. I remember looking out the window and thinking I'm going to be here forever. This is it, I'm alone in this country. I didn't know anyone. It was awful.

That night I didn't move from my bed as I sobbed into the pillow. I didn't sleep a wink. I still had the nasogastric tube and the worker fed me through the night using a large syringe to push the nutritional liquid through the tube and into my stomach.

My parents didn't come until 1 p.m. on the second day, 2 May. I guess they enjoyed a good long sleep-in for the first time in many years without having to worry about me. They planned to stay for ten days to help me bed down at Montreux. Oh, how I longed for their visits those first days. James would come with them but I would never see him. He would sit on the steps outside and someone would keep him company. He was only thirteen. It must have been so hard on him.

A doctor came to see me late on the second day and removed my nasogastric tube. I screamed and cried at the disgusting pain it caused as it was removed. For the first time in two years I didn't have a tube stuck in my nose and it felt weird. But the harsh reality was that I now had to use my lips and mouth to drink the nutritional shakes, which were called Ensure. I had two workers trying to convince me the shakes were safe to drink but I refused. I was in terrible distress. I hadn't put anything in my mouth in a long time and I couldn't bear the thought of doing so. I cried and cried and as time passed my crying got louder and eventually it became a constant scream. That screaming continued day and night for three weeks.

Peggy Claude-Pierre described me as one of the worst cases she'd seen and definitely in the lowest 10 per cent of all admissions. I was very sick, very thin and, to most observers, close to death. By now I was howling so much that everyone, patients and staff, could hear me. Out of utter desperation my workers called Peggy at 1 a.m. and put me on the phone. I didn't stop crying but listened to her for over an hour. 'Everything is going to be OK,' she told me. 'It's safe for the workers to put the drink to your lips.' This routine – my screaming, reassuring calls from Peggy – continued for quite a long time.

By my second night I still hadn't touched food or water. I refused to speak to anyone. I felt like I was having an out of body experience. It felt like I was in a bad dream, a nightmare, and I would wake up any minute and be back in Mum's bed in Melbourne. But it wasn't a dream. I counted the hours, minutes and seconds until I would see my parents the next morning.

The Pink Suite got its ingenious name because all the architraves and skirting boards were painted a dusty pink, and it was where all the acute patients lived when they first arrived. It had two bedrooms – one for me and one for another patient – a living room, kitchen and bath-room. The Grey Suite was at the other end of the Mansion and the attic was up another level. I had the back bed-room which was full of light. It was very spacious and the single bed that sat in the middle seemed so small in the vast space around it. There was also a chest of drawers, a television and a video recorder in the corner of the room. Off my bedroom was a walk-in wardrobe, an ensuite bathroom shared with the other bedroom and a sunroom. There was nothing on the walls but white paint and pink trims.

I rarely left my suite for the first month because I hated Montreux. I wasn't allowed outside because I would try to run away. I don't know where I was planning on running; I just wanted to get away from the place I considered so torturous. I sat on my bed wishing I'd never agreed to go to Montreux.

I eventually got off my bed and took up the habit of standing by the window staring at what was happening around me. I had a view of the amazing garden and lawn that had been established to join the Mansion to the other Montreux house, St Charles, which was bigger than the Mansion and had an even greater presence. It was a mock Tudor-style house built in the 1890s by another wealthy Canadian family.

Like the Mansion, it was divided into small apartments but retained many of its original features both inside and out. It was at the rear of these two houses that they shared gardens, a big grassy area, and a rather large car park to accommodate all the staff. From my vantage point in my room, I could silently observe the movements of the other patients. Without talking to them, I learned their names, where they were from and how long they had been there just by watching and asking my workers the occasional question.

There were times in the Pink Suite that even today make me feel nauseous just thinking about it. There was one day when I was being so influenced by my head that I completely lost control. I was so angry that I picked up a glass vase and threw it, red roses and all, across the room, smashing it into tiny pieces. I then tried to jump out of the sunroom window. My worker grabbed me and as we struggled on the floor I lashed out with my left leg and kicked a large hole in the plasterboard wall. I ran and hid under my bed and stayed there tearing an entire box of tissues into tiny pieces, crying as I did it. Every time I did something like that or kicked holes in the walls, Montreux would have to find someone who was stronger than me. I went through quite a few workers.

Sunday, 19 May 1996

Dear Mum,

Hi! I love you so very much. You're so very special to me. I spoke to you this afternoon but I didn't tell you every-thing on the phone so I thought I would write and tell you. I'm sorry I always waffle on when I'm on the phone but I never get to say what I really want because my stupid anorexia tells me things to say. I hate my anorexia. I just want 'him' to leave me alone.

I want you to know I couldn't survive if anything happened to you. You and Dad are the two most important people to me in my life and I'm just not coping without you both.

Anorexia always scares me, and tells me that bad things will happen and I will lose you. I need to be with you so I can protect you from 'him'. I'm really sorry about all the times I made you cry and feel upset!

I love you and miss you so much.

Love always,

Bronte

Monday, 20 May 1996

Dear Dad,

You're probably so sick of me writing letters to you. Actually I'm not sure if you have got my letters yet. I'll put this letter in with the one I wrote to you yesterday.

I wish I could talk to you and Mum every day but the clinic won't let me. My workers say I have to start thinking of myself and stop worrying about everyone else. I've been trying really hard not to scream. I haven't screamed yet today. I've cried and howled (only a little) but I haven't screamed.

I love and miss you so much. I'm not coping without you. Each day is a struggle and I can't deal with the monster in my head any more.

Take care and say hello to everybody for me.

Love always, hugs and kisses,

Bronte

P.S. Please check that Mum is OK.

Monday, 20 May 1996

Dear Mum,

I'm so bored Mum. I long to have you hug me and to hear your voice. I long to hear and hold Dad also.

Are you safe? Please keep yourself safe. I couldn't bear to lose you and Dad.

I know you think this is the best place for me but I really don't like it here. I'm so scared, lonely and depressed. I cry a lot because I miss you all so much and I just can't deal with this monster in my head. I'm trying so hard.

All my love, hugs and kisses

Bronte

Wednesday, 22 May 1996

I want so much to be normal and get these thoughts, this voice and my fears out of my head. I just want to be happy at home with my family. It seems like it will never happen. I feel like I'll never get better. I'm trying really hard for my Mum and Dad. I'm so scared of losing them! I couldn't go on living without them. I want to do so many things but 'he', the voice in my head, scares me. I don't know what to do.

Thursday, 23 May 1996

I have to get a new toothbrush today because one of the workers touched it and now I'm too scared to use it. They're going to get me a new one but I feel guilty because it's a Sunday and I've made them work today.

I'm so scared of diseases and of losing my Mum and Dad. I try to do things to distract myself but my mind always wanders off onto what 'he' says.

Rituals ruled, or ruined to be more accurate, my life by the time I left for Canada in 1996. These rituals were created by and driven by my anorexia. A typical day was made up of rules and regulations set out by my condition that began the second I woke up and lasted until the second I fell asleep, that's if I slept at all. My day began with me not being allowed to get out of bed until a certain hour, minute or second. If I disobeyed, my anorexia threatened to do all sorts of terrible things, mainly to my family, sometimes to myself and occasionally to society in general. Some threats were general threats such as someone becoming very sick but others were very specific and very frightening. If I disobeyed my thoughts, anorexia would threaten to kill a family member in a car accident, a plane crash or by AIDS. If I disobeyed my thoughts then anorexia would create some natural disaster to wipe out half the planet. The list of shocking, yet creative, ways to help the human race shuffle off this mortal coil went on and on.

The threats weren't just restricted to what time I got out of bed. My head turned a range of everyday things into obsessive rituals such as eating (of course), walking, hand washing, showering, opening doors, watching television, where I sat, what clothes I wore and doing everything to a time frame. If I ate my sandwich in 20 minutes rather than 21 minutes then I would have a thought that Mum would die in a car crash. To avoid the tragedy, I obeyed my head and the more I obeyed, the worse I got.

Sunday, 26 May 1996

I've been at Montreux for three weeks and four days. The time is going so slowly.

I'm so extremely homesick. I'm missing Mum and Dad so much. It hurts so much to be apart from them. I miss Sam, Jordan and James and our dogs, Muffin and Mac. I talk to Mum on Saturdays and Dad on Wednesdays on the phone. I called Mum yesterday and she sounds like she's doing well. I want so much to be home.

I don't like it here at all. I have workers with me 24 hours a day and, believe me, it gets very frustrating. I just want to be left alone but at the same time, I don't want to be alone even in this Pink Suite. They even come to the bathroom with me. There's no shower here so it's a bath or nothing. At first

I couldn't handle it but as time's gone by I've become used to having baths. I get the worker to clean out the bath before I get in because I'm so scared of germs and calories.

I screamed a lot when I first came in but I'm trying really hard not to now. I only scream when I can't handle my head anymore. It hurts when the negative voice gets really loud. I don't know what to do so I scream to try to shut him up. If I'm screaming so loud then I can't hear him as much. 'He' scares me so much. 'He's' always telling me bad things are going to happen. The workers tell me 'he' is a liar and that everyone is safe and that bad things will not happen. I have to ignore him but that's really hard to do. Especially when 'he' has been there for so long.

I feel so fat. I'm fatter than everyone else here. I can't stand living like this. It gets so much that I just can't deal with it any more.

Monday, 27 May 1996

It's about 11 p.m. and I'm just about to get ready for bed so I'm not going to write much. Today was long and hard – just like every other day. I have worried, been lonely, scared, afraid and angry.

I spoke with Dad yesterday and I think he was annoyed with me because I sent him a fax and all I wrote on it was how much I love and miss him and how homesick I am. I miss him and Mum so much and I love them.

I don't like it here.

Tuesday, 28 May 1996

Today was horrible. I spent part of my day crying.

I was meant to go to the movies tonight but Peggy decided that the crowd would be too much for me. She was probably right but I was very disappointed. She said I can probably go tomorrow instead but I'm not sure I believe her. She says I can do things and then doesn't let me do them.

I had a manicure tonight and I'm so frightened because I had a cut on my finger and the woman also had a cut on her finger. I'm sure my cut touched hers and so now I'm going to get a very bad disease. See, I'm too scared to even write the name of the disease. You know what it is! I've been afraid of it all of my life.

Friday, 31 May 1996

It was another awful day today. I cried and screamed a lot too. I even made my carer Shar cry. I'm such a bad person and so selfish. I feel so guilty about all the times I made my family sad. I've ruined their lives.

I planted my garden today. I planted a rose bush, tomatoes, lettuce, peas, sunflowers and carrots. I've been going for drives. I went for a walk and I went to the movies. I enjoy getting out of my room.

Saturday, 1 June 1996

I've now been at Montreux one month today. I hate it more than when I first came here.

My workers say the voice in my head is fighting harder because he knows he's going to lose but I don't know if they can make him go away. He tells me off for

every little thing I do. If I wear certain clothes then
something bad will happen but if I wear other clothes
then bad things will happen also. It's like that with
every little thing I do. He scares me so much. He's
always telling me that Mum and Dad won't be safe
and that bad things will happen to them. He tells me
that Mum and Dad will die. The other fear he always
scares me with is that very bad disease.

Today Peggy came to the house and she was eating
an ice-cream right in front of me. It really scared me
because of the calories. I just wish all my fears would
go away. They hurt so much.

About a month after arriving at Montreux, Peggy
Claude-Pierre called me and announced that my workers
would now be eating in front of me. I was mortified and
refused to be in a room where someone was eating but I
knew I had no choice. Peggy was the voice of authority
at Montreux. She was the boss, much like the principal
of a school that gives out detentions. She had a strong
personality and was a tough disciplinarian, which is why
the patients never disobeyed her. At first I would stand
with my face in the corner so that I didn't have to look at
them eating. My workers would constantly point out that
everyone was still alive when I didn't comply with my
negative mind. This was very hard for me to believe as
my negative mind would constantly move the goalposts
on me and would say, 'Well, I never said they would die
now. It could be any time soon.'

**

Sunday, 2 June 1996

My carers say I'm not allowed to cry any more.
Yesterday when I was crying the next-door neighbour
copied me. Apparently they are really fed up with me
howling and screaming. They have no idea what's
going on in my head. They don't know what it's like
to have mean thoughts in your head ruling you and
screaming at you all day. I can't live like this much
more. I feel bad for distressing people.

By the time I got to the Montreux Clinic there wasn't
a moment when my head wasn't screaming at me for
something and I think, in order to feel in control, my
anorexia became even more ritualistic. I became even
more obsessed with time. I had to time everything I did
and there was a time limit for everything – from drinking
the nutritional supplements to the time it took for each
sip, from the amount of words I could say in an hour to
how long I should brush my teeth. If I didn't do these
things in the set time then my head would threaten me
with the death of a family member. Soon after arriving
my team of workers decided to confiscate my watch.
What a relief for me but what a blow for my anorexia
which decided to hit back. Instead of time being the problem, the amount of times I did things became an issue.

I felt so trapped. As time went by I became angrier and
more tied to my negative mind than ever before. My
anorexia was getting stronger and I was getting weaker.
I didn't do this consciously, of course. I think it was more
that the people at Montreux were trying to back my
anorexia and condition into a corner and like any wild

animal caught in a trap, my anorexia fought back. The workers were now my enemy and I hated them all with a passion. I was being tortured and screaming was my way of coping with it.

I tried to escape many times during those early days but I never succeeded. My workers were too quick and would usually catch me before I could get around the corner, which was no more than 200 metres up the road. I obviously wasn't the only patient who tried to escape so the staff were all pretty quick on their feet.

My care workers would constantly ask for updates on what my head was saying and what the threats were. This was really hard to do because my head threatened me with the latest tragedy if I told them. I was so tired of it all that I started to tell them what was happening. I wanted someone to make it stop.

Monday, 3 June 1996

Another day living with anorexia – another day being ruled by him. I was up til 4 a.m. crying. It really wore me out so I slept in until 10 a.m. today. I have to take so many tablets. I take 12 fibre pills, two Docusate (for constipation), two calcium tablets and one multi-vitamin pill per day.

There is no way I would be here if I'd known how horrible it was going to be. I feel so afraid and alone. I'm not sure how to deal with all these feelings.

I spent an hour sitting in the wardrobe trying to escape the voice in my head. But 'he' always follows me no matter where I go. I can't escape 'him'. 'He's' everywhere surrounding me and torturing me. My carers tell me 'he's' a bully and to not listen to 'him' but it's a lot harder than it sounds. Sometimes I get myself worked up into such a state that I go totally off my face. I start to scream and I can't stop.

I had a long talk with Peggy today, which helped me. I gave her my list of things I'm afraid of and also a list of the foods that would be OK! I'm not sure when I'll start to eat but I think it's when I'm ready. I don't think I could put the food in my mouth. It would just be too hard.

I'm going to try really hard not to scream. I'm going to try to think about all the other people in the house. Today has been hard and I'm glad it's over.

Tuesday, 4 June 1996

I've moved to the attic. I like it up here much better than in the Pink Suite. I have my own little room with a pitched roof and there is a shower above the bath here which I'm so happy about!

I made a deal with Peggy that if I didn't cry for three days I could move to a room in the attic, which had the prized possession of a shower instead of a bath. She agreed and I stopped crying. My new room was tiny and cosy. The floor was tiled in orange terracotta, it had a peaked ceiling and, as it was on the third floor, my little window overlooked the ocean and mountains. I stayed in the attic for four months. It was here I went onto food.

I started to get out of the house more. I would go for short walks to the grand old Lieutenant Governor's Mansion, which was just down the road. I would go down to Victoria's quaint inner harbour in the evenings but, as this was still very difficult for me because of my phobias, I would always have two workers with me. I began to visit Irma, a wonderful German art teacher who came to the clinic twice a week and worked with us in a little studio in the basement of the Mansion. My head made me feel guilty about these visits because they were considered a luxury.

I still didn't sleep well and I would often try to sleep on the floor without a blanket or pillow because that's all I believed I deserved. I wasn't allowed to stay on the floor and quite often Peggy would come to the clinic at all hours of the night to help my workers get me to understand I was worthy of a bed, worthy of sleep and worthy of my snacks.

I had two room-mates in the attic – Sophie from the United States and Aviva from Israel. I was always trying to do something to make their day better so on my walks to the Lieutenant Governor's Mansion I would pick two of the most beautiful roses I could find on the property and take them home to these sick girls. Little did I know that I could be fined $500 for taking a rose.

Tuesday, 6 August 1996
A Poem

Dark and cold
All on my own.
Him inside
Gaining control.
No longer two
We then became One.
Where did her life go? How was it lost?
She didn't see,
All she needed was him.

His world now was hers,
A world in which freedom no longer existed,
Happiness didn't live and smiling didn't survive.
No one could enter as he was there.
A friend who promised her much love and comfort
Who has more power as time goes by.
No trust and belief except for with him.
That dark shadowing voice that comes from within,
So strong, so real, so loud and so clear.
The outside world misty, she can't see or hear.
This is her life, she has so long for lived,
Her life now trying to exist.
For this is the way she feels she must live.

Wednesday, 14 August 1996

I'm feeling trapped inside my head. 'He' is really loud and yelling at me a lot. I'm so scared of gaining weight. I feel so fat and ugly. I can't stand my big body. I don't even fit into my clothes anymore. I feel like I have to hang my head in shame because that way no one would have to look at my ugly face. I'm not allowed to do anything because my head doesn't allow me.

'He' gave me a heap of trouble for opening my mouth to eat. I don't deserve to eat! I don't need it and I don't want it! In fact, I totally despise food. I can't stand the sight of myself.

The tedious process of eating a snack took up most of my day. I had difficulty holding a fork so my worker's hand would rest on mine and help guide the food to my mouth. I felt overwhelming guilt doing this all by myself.

Friday, 23 August 1996

I've been at the clinic for almost four months now –
the hardest four months of my life. I really don't like it
here and I want to go home. Sometimes when I'm
having an OK day, I think it's not so bad here. But then
when I'm having a day like I did today, I absolutely
despise this place. I don't like my care workers; they
annoy me.

I'm eating food now. I didn't eat solid food for two-
and-a-half months; all I was having were the [Ensure]
shakes.

Life was very much about restraint at Montreux. There
were rules I had to obey to protect me from my 'head'.
At the time my anorexia was so out of control I didn't see
it that way. Instead I thought everyone was mean and
nasty trying to wean me off my safety blanket – my
phobias, rituals and the need to obey anorexia.

I had a team of five or so carers who would work
around the clock. One would arrive at 8 a.m. and stay
until 4 p.m. and another would arrive for the evening
shift which finished at midnight. My evening worker
would come and stay until 8 a.m.

I knew when a worker wasn't knowledgeable about
anorexia and I knew when they were scared of the illness. I didn't like these workers. I felt unsafe with them.
It wasn't that they were bad in any way. On the contrary,
most of them were lovely. Their inexperience made it
easier for me to eat them up and spit them out in a
second. Often they fled in tears.

There were times in my acute stage of treatment where my workers would have to physically restrain me from acting out my rituals. This would usually end with me in tears, panicked about what would happen next. When I brushed my teeth I had to rinse my mouth out six times for the six people in my family. If I did less than six rinses then a certain number of people would die. If I did it more then we would all die. My workers could see these rituals and would try to stop me following through with them. One time my carer Cindy actually put her hand over my mouth and stopped me rinsing more than once. We had a Mexican standoff until I eventually moved. It got harder as my head got angrier with my carer and me. Eventually, Cindy and the others started to win. Even though I had the urge to follow through on the rituals, I now had the strength to stop myself.

At first, challenges, such as new food, were planned. Knowing in advance freaked me out and gave me time to mull over the challenge and create ways for getting out of it. My workers agreed that I was better off not knowing when things were going to change. Challenges were then continually sprung on me to confront and shock my fears.

Saturday, 24 August 1996

I had to stop writing last night because Peggy called to tell me to go to sleep. I did because nobody dares disobey Peggy.

The voice in my head got much louder during the first few months I was here at Montreux. 'He' was so loud and so mean I didn't think I could go on anymore but Peggy helped me through. 'He's' still extremely loud now but I'm just not allowed to listen.

Some things are very slowly becoming easier. 'He' still tells me really mean stuff but not as often as 'he' used to. I think if 'he' had the chance he would probably rule my whole day but the people here don't give 'him' that chance. It frustrates me so much. They tell me what to do and how to do it all day long. They tell me I only have 20 minutes to eat! How unfair is that! I hate being bossed around by anyone but at the same time I hate making decisions for myself and I hate the thought of taking care of myself!

I don't think I deserve a place in this world. I don't feel I deserve anything and I certainly don't deserve to be at this clinic. I'm not even sick enough to be here. I'm so much fatter than every other person here. I wish I could be my goal weight of 37 kg. I have no idea what I weigh now – my mind tells me I weigh about 60 kg or 70 kg. I wouldn't be surprised if that were my weight. I'm so much fatter than when I first got here.

I don't cry much any more. I only cry when 'he' is really loud and mean.

Sunday, 1 September 1996

I moved to a new house today. It's called St Charles. I'm on the second level right next to Peggy's office. I share with Aviva, my old room-mate from the attic. We're in a studio apartment that has everything except the bathroom all in the one room. It's very small for two people and our beds are so close together that we have a privacy screen between us. I'm lucky as my bed is next to the window that has a really nice view of the ocean and mountains. You can even see the United States from here – it's that close.

Moving to the adjoining St Charles house was a big step in the right direction as St Charles was the place you went to when you were doing a little better. I shared a studio apartment with one of my previous room-mates, Aviva, and it was very cramped. I had neighbours in the rooms on either side of me. One room was Peggy's office and the other room was occupied by Charlie, one of the other patients.

Charlie was in his late teens when I met him. He was short and sweet with mousy-brown hair and blue eyes. Charlie had a baby face and seemed a very odd English character to me at the time. He would not only teach me how to juggle but would become one of my very dear friends and would ultimately have a hand in helping me fight my fears.

Thursday, 5 September 1996

It's about midnight on a Friday. I'm tired but I'm not going to sleep. Sometimes anorexia makes deals with me and will let me do certain things in return for not doing other things, like sleep.

It rained all day long which was depressing in itself. I woke up to a worker I didn't like at all but an hour later a good worker arrived so that made me feel better.

I still don't like it here and I still want to go home so badly. I spoke to Mum tonight for half an hour. It was so nice to hear her voice. I miss her and Dad immensely. She was telling me heaps of funny stories and making me laugh so hard! She is such an awesome Mum.

Friday, 6 September 1996

I think Peggy couldn't call me tonight because she was just too busy. It's stressing me out! I didn't talk to her all day. I miss her a lot too! She means a lot to me even though I don't know her all that well. She helps me feel so safe. When I'm with her I feel like nothing can hurt me or anyone I care about. It's almost as if she's protecting everyone around me too! It's amazing what just one person can do! She saved me from dying (mentally) and she's trying to take 'him' away from me. As much as 'he' hurts me, it's really painful to have 'him' dragged away from me! Who am I without anorexia? What will there be? No one, nothing. Probably even more emptiness than I feel now! I can't even comprehend the thought of living a normal life in the real world and being happy and not scared and ruled by a monster in my head!

Peggy yells at me a lot, especially when I don't do what she tells me. 'He' is so loud and I would rather do what 'he' says than what she says. Some days I just loathe Peggy! Other days I just really miss her because she can't be with me 24 hours a day. Even though I'm angry with her most of the time I still want to talk to her constantly!

Peggy became involved in my treatment very early on. She was almost like the leader of my team. I had carers who would be with me all day and night to look after me and make sure I stuck to my program. I would then go to sessions twice a week to see my counsellors who would try to talk about my issues such as my fears, food and obsessive behaviour.

Kirsten, Peggy's oldest daughter, was my first counsellor at Montreux. Tall with dark mysterious eyes and jet-black hair, she looked like her mother but was the complete opposite to her sister, Nicole. Kirsten was the first of the two sisters to become sick with anorexia. When she got better, Nicole got sick. Kirsten was softly spoken and gentle. She was an introvert and had a constant calmness about her.

Peggy would call or visit me everyday, usually to calm a storm whipped up by my anorexia. I became very dependent on her and tended to put her on a pedestal, as did every other patient at Montreux. There were times when I wouldn't listen to my care workers but I would listen to Peggy. She had a calmness to her that was endearing when she wasn't wearing her disciplinarian hat. She would tell me how much stronger she was than my anorexia and that she was not going to let my illness win. She promised me she would never give up on me. Her strength and support became less frequent, though, as she became busier. I became upset that the one person I trusted had left me. This helped me to lean on my care workers more and to trust other people. I began to let other people into my world and realised that Peggy was not the only person who could help me.

Saturday, 7 September 1996

I'm such a little annoying brat! I feel like everyone here hates me so much. They're just pretending to like me because that's what they get paid to do. I don't want anyone's help. I'm just fine on my own! I can look after myself.

I have counselling sessions with Kirsten on Mondays and Wednesdays and I see Diana on Fridays. I tell my counsellors what a waste of time I am every time I see them. They don't seem to believe me but I'm determined to prove it to them! I feel like I'm too FAT to be here and that I'm using a space that some really sick, sad, dying and unhappy person could be using. I'm so selfish taking up space here. They don't even recognise the changes I have made.

When I first came here I was so afraid of food I couldn't even look at it! Now I eat a meal plan everyday and I eat at the same time as the other people eat AND in the same room!! Many of my phobias and fears have lessened in four and a half months! There are still millions and trillions of things 'he' makes me do or things 'he' makes me scared of but I have to try to ignore him! It's SO, SO, SO, HARD. I don't think I can bear to live in this hell much longer!

Sunday, 8 September 1996

It's Sunday morning about 8.30. I just finished eating a muffin and I drank a white grape juice too! I'm still sitting in bed, not really wanting to get up and face the day. It's just so much easier to stay in bed because then I wouldn't have to feel guilty about going out.

I have been out so much since I came here. I go shopping a lot but the malls are so small compared to the ones at home. I go to the beach but the beaches here are not as nice as they are at home.

I do things here at the clinic too. I have an Educational Program – which I absolutely despise – every weekday! I also do art three times a week and have *piano lessons on Thursday. I get weighed on Mondays and Thursdays which I don't like at all.*

Tuesday, 10 September 1996

I've decided that I hate my life and myself.

I hate Montreux.

I hate anorexia.

I hate Bronte.

I hate being sad and I hate feeling happy only every now and then.

I'm sick of having to put up with the crap anorexia dishes out to me. Day after day after day. It's never-ending. Sometimes I feel like I'm running around in circles bashing my head against a brick wall. I know I've made changes since I've been here but I just feel stuck in a rut. Every minute seems like an eternity to me.

Mum will be here in 11 days. I can't believe I will actually have her here. I haven't seen her in four and a half months, that's way too long. I miss her and Dad so much. I'm afraid she won't like me anymore because I'm a little bit more outspoken now than when I was at home. People didn't like me before I got sick, now they will hate me even more.

It's 12.45 a.m. and Peggy didn't call me tonight. She used to call, or come and see me, just about every night. But suddenly she's too busy with all the other patients. I feel so angry with myself when she doesn't call. I love talking to her because she makes me feel so safe. Yet at the same time, I'm absolutely petrified of her. She yells at me if I don't eat my food, she yells at me for listening to my head. The only reason I eat is because I'm afraid of Peggy. The only reason I do what

I'm told is because I'm afraid of Peggy. The only reason I don't cry is because I'm afraid of Peggy yelling at me. It appears that everything I do is for the wrong reason. In fact, it seems like everything I do is wrong these days. No one thinks I try hard enough.

I've decided that I want to become a mute. I don't want to speak to anyone here ever again. I'm going to test it out, starting tomorrow. I'll let you know how it goes. I hate the fact that I have to have a carer with me 24 hours a day. I hate it with a passion. I want some time on my own even if it's just an hour. I need my own space.

I'm so mad that Peggy didn't bother to call me. She hates me now and I don't blame her. Talking to me everyday for four months would probably send me around the bend. I just feel as if she thinks I don't need her help. Maybe she's right. Maybe I don't need anyone here. All I need is my family. I need to be home. I want to be HOME. I miss my home!

Monday, 16 September 1996

Bronte is:

Mean

Undeserving

Ugly

Worthless

Nasty

Selfish

Horrible

Unwanted

Unloved

Bad
This is how I feel today.

Wednesday, 18 September 1996

Hi Dad. Here's a diary entry just for you. I couldn't have asked for a more perfect father. You gave up your life, your world, for me. If it weren't for you, I doubt I would be sitting here writing in this diary today. You gave me a reason to get up and live every day. You never gave up on me even when others threw in the towel. You never left me alone, and put up with all my crap. I know that most of the time, you were probably so frustrated and angry with me, as I was with life. I'm sorry for hurting you and the rest of the family so much. Just look how much anorexia has changed our lives and turned them totally upside down. I know how much it has affected your lives and I feel so bad for that. But just think, I will be coming home one day (hopefully soon) and we'll be together again, but it won't be like it used to be. We will be together, living a life of happiness without the dreadful monster in my head controlling me. And you won't have to throw Weet-Bix and orange juice on me ever again. Just look now, I can eat food on my own. I don't have to have someone hand feeding me.

Saturday, 21 September 1996

Mum and Aunty Bronte arrived today. It was so wonderful to see them again. I can't wait to spend more time with them.

I've been reading through my notepad and found this poem I wrote about six weeks ago. I know you'll be able to figure out what it means and I know that you will understand it.

FALLING
Huddled so silent,
Insignificant yet not,
She sits cornered with fear,
Consumed with pain by him.
FALLING
Look deep inside,
The child is there,
She may seem small,
Desperately needing to leave,
Disappear from the big bad world.
FALLING
A tear is shed,
No one need care,
He has her at last,
Caught in his web.
FALLING
The child is weak,
Too afraid and too lost,
All hope gone,
So the stronger he fought!
FALLING
She is caught at last,
Just before she fell,
Her spirit reborn,
May she wake well.

Thursday, 10 October 1996

So much has happened since I last wrote. My Mum has been and gone, Peggy has been on her European lecture tour and anorexia has been up to its usual tricks.

It seems like I'm going backwards. I'm feeling very lonely. Peggy isn't talking to me very much any more. Ever since she's been away she thinks I don't need her – so obviously I don't. Therefore I just won't speak to her ever again. I'm a pretty stubborn person and I'm so mad at her right now that I can't even describe my anger! I feel so trapped here. I'm forced to eat! I absolutely despise FOOD! I don't know how they think they are going to fix me!

Sometimes life's just too much to deal with! I'm so angry that I could just scream. The only place I can get my anger out is on paper. I'm sorry you're the one I have to vent it on but you're the only source that listens and doesn't answer back.

So much is racing around and around in my head. I don't want to wake up to tomorrow. Please give me strength to deal with anorexia and fight it again tomorrow. What would my life consist of without anorexia? Would it be bliss or would it be empty? I couldn't know because I don't remember not having 'him' in my head.

Sometimes I feel like I'm going to go insane here. I get told to try that little bit harder – be that little bit braver. Well, what I would like to know is how brave can one be? I was extremely brave when I went with Cindy – my team leader – to get the top part of my ear pierced. I'm so scared of what disease I've caught because I got it pierced!

I absolutely loved my visit with Mum and Aunty Bronte. I took them shopping and we just hung out and talked and talked and talked. Mum bought me heaps of stuff. That made me feel bad because I *already feel like I have way too many clothes. I don't deserve new things. Mum bought me a watch.*

Have to go.

Cindy was my first team leader, overseeing my other five or so workers. She knew my anorexia inside out and knew what would set it off and what I could cope with. She made sure the whole team was on the same wavelength. She had just returned from a trip to Australia and was quite an Aussie fan when we met so we hit it off instantly.

This Canadian had a hint of hippy about her. She was in her late twenties, tall with long wavy reddish pink hair and newly married. She had a vibrancy about her that I didn't see in everyone working at Montreux. She was so strong with my very vocal and, at times, violent anorexia. She was tough on my condition and was adamant about me not following through with my rituals and not listening to my 'head'. She didn't let up for one second which caused me so much grief at the time.

To cope with my pain Cindy would drive me down to the beach and tell me to let it all out by screaming at the top of my lungs. I did and I would feel better. She stayed with me throughout my acute stage at Montreux. We had many adventures together. I even shared in the adventure of her first pregnancy. She had her beautiful little girl, Pheonix, and moved onto a new stage of her life. I was very sad to see her go.

Colin was one of my counsellors and Shar was one of my workers. Shar was a new worker at Montreux when she was assigned to my team, or, as it was more often known, my 'case' as if I were a criminal with a team of detectives working around the clock. Standing 5 foot nothing, with big brown eyes and bobbed brown hair, Shar was gentle and kind and had a distinct motherly presence about her, probably because she was mum to a gorgeous little boy and girl. Shar was a dancer before joining the clinic and although she had experienced some training, she knew very little about the illness. We learned together. She became my team leader after Cindy left.

Colin was quite a character. He really was a frustrated film-maker who somehow ended up working at Montreux. He was in his late twenties, tall, blond, blue-eyed and gorgeous. All the girls went weak at the knees at the sight of Colin.

Friday, 11 October 1996

Today was better than yesterday, which wasn't hard. To begin with it was sunny for once. Amazing! I was still really angry with Peggy all day today for not talking to me! I avoided her the whole day.

Saturday, 19 October 1996

I went for two walks today. They weren't really long walks though as my workers don't let me go too far in case I might be trying to burn off fat.

I hate this place! I miss my Mum and Dad and Muffin the dog so much. I don't think I can stand it much more. I just want to go home. Peggy hates me even more than I hate her. Everyone here thinks I'm annoying and pretending to be sick. I feel like I shouldn't let anyone get close to me. I'm very angry inside but I don't want to let anyone know how I feel.

I have been going to Educational Program (they call
it EP here) as well as piano lessons and still painting
with Irma. I also enjoy listening to all kinds of music
and sometimes get into writing letters. It can get very
boring here and very frustrating.

I hate the way they make me eat! I'm so huge and
I'm getting bigger everyday. I hate food and I don't want
to eat ever, ever again. I want to run away. I don't know
who I'm angrier at – the clinic, anorexia or me? I feel so
TRAPPED! Life is so, so unfair. But then no one said it
would be easy. I'm so scared inside and I feel so alone. I
don't even have Peggy to help me any more. She calls
me about every three days. I'm just another number.

I forgot to mention I'm learning how to juggle but
I'm not very good!

Sunday, 10 November 1996
Bronte's Dream List

To be happy.

To save all the dying children in third world countries.

To cure all the disease in the world.

To take everyone's pain away.

For there to be sunshine every day of the year.

To be an animation artist for Disney.

Ride the Viper at Magic Mountain with my Dad.

Travel to Germany, Paris, Greece and Italy.

To be a television news reporter.

To go home and have my own apartment.

To go on a train ride through the Rocky Mountains
with my family.

For the monster in my head to go away and leave me
alone.

Saturday, 16 November 1996

I've been at Montreux for seven long, long months. The
following poem is how I'm feeling at this point in time.

So lost and afraid in a world of her own,
She must defend herself, do it alone.
So many years of being afraid,
Living in shadows,
Behind closed doors.

Unloved, unwanted, un-needed, alone,
The fear too great to conquer the world.
Run away, hide,
But no place to hide except deep inside.

No where in the world to call my own.

Home, so far out of reach,
Beyond comprehension of normalcy and peace,
At war inside, when will it end,
Her spirit, self, being, should she fight for and defend.

Dictated by the voice inside,
Needing yet not allowing to cry.

So lost and afraid in a world of her own.
Her time in the world too much overgrown.

Sunday, 1 December 1996

Right now I'm having a really rough time with my
head. I'm silent most of the day and cry quite a bit too.
The voice in my head is still really loud and I don't know

how to fight back. I hate feeling scared, sad and alone most of the time. I miss my family immensely and ache inside to be with them. I miss my bed at home. I miss my house. But I don't miss the hospital bed! And I don't miss the TUBE. I want to be free. I want to be happy but I don't think I'll ever be. When I feel sad like I do right now and can't see an end to the pain, I no longer feel like trying! Everything feels like it's just too much for me right now!

It's very late at night so I'd better scoot. Lots of love to the whole world that I wish I could fix!

Monday, 2 December 1996

Today was a BAD day and I'm not sure really how to describe it. It seems like it has lasted forever and I'm glad it's finally over. It was so, so hard.

I feel so angry and tormented inside. I feel lost, alone and scared. I'm being beaten up inside my head; I just want a break from 'him' – the voice in my head. I want to be home with my family and friends and to no longer be his prisoner. I want to go back and just be me. No voices coming with me. I can't imagine 'him' not being in my head. I think Peggy thinks 'he's' gone but 'he' hasn't. Maybe she'll let me go home. Who knows?

Tuesday, 3 December 1996

Tonight I just cried, cried and cried so much that now I have a headache. I'm not really tired so I'm trying to write until I do feel sleepy. I feel so empty inside right now and so unloved and distant from the rest of the world. I feel so alone with 'him' just screaming and yelling at me. 'He's' so mean but 'he's' been there so long.

I haven't really been going out lately. I just feel too bad about myself, and life, to be seen in public. I just don't feel like being a part of life!

Thursday, 5 December 1996

At last, some good news. Mum rang to say she is coming to visit me in three weeks time. I can't wait to see her again. It's a shame the rest of the family can't make it but at least I will have Mum with me once again.

Sunday, 8 December 1996

Another long and hard day – aren't they all? It feels like it's gone on and on and on and on! It's nearly Christmas! Only 17 days to go and only 16 days until Mum arrives. I can't wait to see her again but I do wish Dad was coming with her. I miss him terribly.

As much as I miss home and my family, I don't want to be there. It's all very confusing. I sort of feel very alone.

I've been having bad days lately. I'm so SCARED. I have to get weighed tomorrow and I'm scared that I've gained weight.

I just spoke with Peggy. She called to say she loves me and that I sounded stronger. Right! Like I believe that one. I don't feel stronger but I didn't tell her that.

It's late and I'm tired but I'm scared to go to sleep because I've been having bad dreams lately.

It frightened me to think about home because I was so sick when I was there. I associated home with anorexia.

I thought, 'If I go home, will things be the same, will I get sick again and end up in hospital living a miserable life?' Home wasn't just my family. It was everything – an entire place, Melbourne, Australia. It was all way too scary and there were too many question marks. My emotions were swirling around in complete conflict. I wanted to be with my family but I hated the thought of being home.

Monday, 9 December 1996

Well, today is only half over and I already feel totally awful. I woke up at 5.30 a.m. I've been having really bad nightmares lately which haven't been helping my sleep. I wrote Christmas cards for a while and even did some doodling until Shar arrived. I ate, had a shower and made my bed . . . blah, blah, blah.

I spotted Peggy just as I was about to be weighed today. I wanted to avoid her so I asked Margaret [who was doing the weighing] to hurry up. I was half successful. Just as I was leaving, Peggy came in but at least she didn't weigh me. Phew! I like to hug her though. She is so nice to hug.

I was supposed to move up to the top of St Charles house today but Peggy couldn't organise it. I totally understand as she's the busiest person in the world! I don't know how she can understand anorexia so well. Sometimes I don't think she does understand me. She thinks I'm well, I'm sure of it. Well, if that's what she thinks then I want to know why she's not letting me go home? I don't like it here not one bit AT ALL!

I've been in this clinic for seven months and nine days, which is a long time to be away from my family. I feel so weird looking around this room. This is my home but it doesn't feel like a real home at all. I don't feel like I belong anywhere. I feel so out of place in this country. It's cold and wet outside so I feel like it's July but I have to keep reminding myself that it is DECEMBER. It just doesn't feel like Christmas especially without my family. I feel so EMPTY, ALONE and ISOLATED. It's a horrible feeling.

I had a counselling session with Kirsten today, which was rather distressing. She told me that I have to go out to eat with her. There is no way in the world I'm going to do that! I absolutely refuse. She decided a couple of weeks ago that I was to eat on the couch instead of eating on my bed where I felt safe. It's so hard to change my routine, it makes everything else feel so much worse.

Thursday, 26 December 1996

What a day. What a Christmas. I was going to write about it yesterday but I was too tired from the whole Christmas day thing and worn out emotionally from my presents. I kept telling Mum I didn't want anything for Christmas except my whole family. Everyone had me believing that my Mum was the only person who was coming and that was good enough for me. Christmas morning came around and I got all my presents from the clinic. Then Mum called me to tell me she'd meet me in the conference room. She said my Christmas present was very big and heavy and she didn't have enough paper to wrap it up. So at 10 a.m. I met Mum downstairs. I opened the door and sitting in a row on the couch were James, Samantha, Dad and Jordan. It was the most incredible Christmas present I've ever received!

**

Late 1996 was the longest winter I've ever felt but one thing that brightened it for me was the surprise visit of my family for Christmas. They saved me from a state of monotony and perpetual sadness where my days consisted of refusing to leave my room, refusing to socialise and asking to go home. I felt like a part of me was ignited and brought to life when my family arrived. I was still only living for them at this stage; not for myself.

We experienced a snowstorm like no other that winter. It started on Christmas Day and its after-effects stayed with us for the next three weeks. It doesn't usually snow in Victoria as the town sits on the Pacific coast and is usually quite mild (it was considered mild at just 2°C). The normally pleasant weather attracts older Canadians looking to retire in the former trading port, turned naval base, turned sleepy provincial capital. The city's burghers sold all the snow ploughing equipment years ago as they figured they would never use it.

The snow in the winter of '96 was waist high, cutting off access to all roads (oh, if only the burghers had kept those ploughs). It looked beautiful, especially to us Australians, but the reality was that we became prisoners of the weather. Me trapped at the clinic and my family at the hotel in town, an hour's walk away. Despite the conditions, my family escaped their hotel to trudge through the snow, arriving wet-legged and tired everyday, to see me. Eventually, we lost all power and heat and no one could sail or fly in or out of the island so food supplies became short. A state of emergency was declared and the army came in to help out. That was my first 'mild' Canadian winter.

Friday, 27 December 1996

It's the day after the day after Christmas. I've got the flu – or something – so I'm not feeling too dandy. I hope I don't give it to my family. I don't want them to get sick while they're here!

It's been snowing for three days straight and I'm getting tired of it. The snow is about knee deep now. You know, it's never meant to snow in this part of Canada.

I saw Mum, Dad and Sam today which was really nice. I felt a bit stressed afterwards but I talked to Peggy which made me feel a bit better after that.

Mum and Dad videoed me juggling. I really don't like being videotaped but if that's what they want then I'll do it as I would do anything for them. I love them to pieces. I can't believe they travelled halfway across the world to be with me. It really means a lot to me. I feel like I'm not good enough to be with them. I feel like I should make the most of the time I have with them while they're here but at the same time it's so overwhelming seeing them all at once, and it has been so long since I've seen them. I'm feeling really guilty now about stuff.

1997

Thursday, 2 January 1997

I woke up in a filthy mood today. I didn't sleep well and I just wasn't ready to face another day.

I got weighed this morning, which wasn't fun at all. I also went to the movies and met Jordan and Dad. It's been so long since I've gone to a movie with Dad. It was really neat to have him there, and Jordan held my hand. They helped me feel safe. It's been so strange seeing them all again. I don't remember a time when we were all together like this. We were hardly ever at home at the same time! We basically lived our own separate lives except when we slept in the same house.

I have lots of thoughts spinning around in my mind. Lots of ideas and thoughts that 'he' says to me! I feel like things are getting really tough.

I'm going to sleep now. I'll be 18 tomorrow. Not that it really matters or that anyone really cares. I know there were times when I said I didn't want to make it to 18 – but I do want to now.

Friday, 3 January 1997

Dear Mum, Dad, Jordan, Sam and James,
I want to thank you all so much for making my Christmas wish come true this year. My exact words,

if I remember correctly, were, 'I just want my Mum to wrap my family up and bring them to me for Christmas. I don't want anything else.' It meant so much to me that you all came so far to be with me to give me a nice Christmas.

Sometimes when you guys were here I had to pinch myself or slap myself across the face so I would know that I wasn't dreaming. I was hugging you, holding my Dad's hand! You can't believe how nice that felt for me!

I hope I gave you some happiness in return. I really enjoyed being able to go out and about to spend some time with you guys. I don't remember the last time we were together and actually spent this much time together.

Well, my birthday is finally over! It's just after midnight. It doesn't feel any different being 18 and I can't even drive yet! Oh well, plenty of time ahead!

I'll miss you lots. My heart is aching for you already, and you haven't even gone anywhere yet! I love you all more than the stars, moons, planets and sun in the sky.

Bronte

Wednesday, 8 January 1997

My family left today. I'm feeling very sad. Samantha left me a note in my pocket saying that my smile looked good on me and I should wear it more often. Dad was so upset that he couldn't say goodbye.

Monday, 13 January 1997

Christmas is over and so is my birthday. My family has gone home and I'm left here once again. It was really neat to see them all but at the same time a very scary concept for me! It's so wonderful they could see me but the biggest drawback was they had to leave again. It was so nice to be able to hug and talk to them instead of yelling at them. They were so nice to me and when I saw them I realised how much I want to be with them and have nothing in my head bossing me around. To be free from that, I wonder what that feels like? To be able to go out to do whatever, eat whatever and not feel guilty or think twice about it! I don't believe that will ever happen. I want it to so badly. I want to be free so much.

I've been at the clinic for almost nine months! It feels a lot longer than that. I want to go home so badly. I don't belong here. I just don't fit in! I feel so lost and empty right now. I miss my family already and they've only just left. I especially miss my Dad. I know that we'll be together one day soon and I can't wait until we are.

January 1997 was a very hard month for me. After my family returned to Australia, I was angry and felt very alone. On top of this I was confronted with an awful challenge. I was told that I was to start eating out for breakfast. I had only just become comfortable with my very plain daily meal plan at the clinic and then this happened.

Breakfast was a small portion of muffin loaf (a secret Montreux recipe) and a Peggy mug of white grape juice (a Peggy mug was an ordinary white China mug used to measure my food). The dreaded morning arrived and so did Shar and Colin, who were sent to take me out to eat. I refused to go. I was told that I had no choice and I was asked if I thought I would ever be ready to challenge myself. I scoffed at this question and answered haughtily, which is how I spoke to most people at the time, 'No, of course I won't.' I refused to put my shoes on.

My negative mind was out of control on this particular morning, more so than usual due to what lay ahead. My shoes, a pair of blue and grey Vans, were pushed onto my feet and tied up. I stood there as still as a statue and refused to move. My two care workers took one arm each and dragged me down four flights of stairs to their car. We were off.

We went to a little English-style teahouse in Oak Bay, a suburb known for the above average age of its residents. The teahouse had the distinct smell of 'old' about it. The walls were covered in floral motifs and much to my disgust the floral tablecloths had been turned over for the morning breakfast run rather than washed from the previous day. I refused to order. I felt that by ordering I was somehow choosing to eat out when in reality I had been dragged there.

Shar and Colin, who were trying to do the right thing, ordered for me and when the food arrived I refused to eat. I sat there for two hours. One hour was spent refusing to eat while the other was spent coming to the realisation that I had no choice so I actually began to eat the muffin at a painfully slow rate. I yelled at Shar and Colin and told them how much I hated them and Peggy for doing this to me. This was something I'd always felt bad about when I was in a more 'rational' place, as it was not in my nature to be so cruel. When anorexia took over, my behaviour often went against my true nature.

These struggles between my condition and my support team at Montreux went on for months. The more they pushed my anorexia, the more negative and nasty I became. I went into a black hole and didn't see how I was ever going to get myself out of it. Having my snacks out became a daily event. New restaurants were added to the list but I still had similar food at each place. I would cry and scream in the restaurants. The more I did this, the more I had to eat out. I felt like I was dying inside. My head was so out of control and everything I had worked on up until this point seemed to be thrown out the window. The pain was endless and I felt like I couldn't keep fighting against my head. Looking back, I must have been well known around the little Victorian restaurants and cafés for my vocal protests to let everyone know that I didn't want to be there.

Saturday, 18 January 1997

I don't like it here at Montreux at all!! Full of anger. I want to go home. Feel lost, alone. Nobody here cares. I'm unimportant. Better now. Fat. Ugly. Ever fatter. They can't help me. I will not take their help. I will not ask. I feel selfish and useless. They have no clue about what I think. I absolutely do not believe them at all and I think they are all a BUNCH of liars. I would hope they weren't but I'm sad to say that sometimes, not all the time though, they are.

I know this is an ANGRY entry. I was trying to use this diary for good things, thoughts and feelings but I needed to vent my anger somewhere.

I'm just so sorry for everything. I feel guilty and bad. I know I'm a horrible person.

Sunday, 19 January 1997

Help me, what can I do? I can't live here one more day. I've decided I don't want to eat one more thing. I hate food. I'm getting fatter day by day. It's not fair. But then as Peggy would say, 'Life's not fair'. How true. And speaking of Peggy, she's in Hawaii for five weeks and I haven't spoken to her for forever. She didn't do what she said she would but that didn't surprise me because she never keeps promises. She said she'd be in close contact and she would call three times a week. Mega lies! Anyway, I don't care. Actually I do. But I wished I didn't because I know she doesn't give two hoots. She doesn't really care about anything that I do. Sometimes I feel like I basically run my own ship yet at other times feel I have no control over it.

I miss my family like crazy – I'm going insane without them.

Monday, 20 January 1997

The snow has melted although I still find the odd lump every now and then. It was so weird snowing here because Victoria is meant to be the warmest place in Canada. So much for that theory! It's been a little bit warmer lately with the temperature reaching 7°C. I can now step outside without my coat!

Sam has gone back to university. I envy her studying. I'll never have that opportunity because of my anorexia. It's not fair. I'll continue to fight as I miss school (sometimes) and I crave to learn.

Thursday, 30 January 1997

I'm hurting so badly inside. I'm so confused and angry and upset. My head is beating me up. I feel so fat and need to lose lots and lots of weight. I don't want workers with me any more. I can take care of myself. My worker Shar went away for a couple of weeks. I'm scared without her. I feel like she is my backbone.

Monday, 17 February 1997

I hate it here. I hate it here. I hate it here. I hate it here. I hate it here. I hate it here. As time goes by I hate it even more.

It's been raining a lot which really depresses me. I want winter to finish so we can enjoy some of the sun that Australia is having right now. I miss my family so much. Every time I call them I feel so bad because I'm unhappy and they notice it too! I try to be happy for them but I guess they can tell.

Peggy comes home next Monday and has promised to work really hard with me. She said she would even be my team leader but I don't believe her. I don't believe anyone around here very much. I think most of them lie. I know they're lying to me about my weight. They say that I'm not putting on weight but I know that's so not true.

Friday, 7 March 1997

Some nights I lie in bed and look at my family photos and wish I had their arms around me, hugging me and holding me all night when I'm so scared. I wonder what they're planning to do for Mum's birthday? I can't believe she'll be 41. She seems so much younger.

I'll tell you a funny story about expressing feelings. While Peggy was away she would call sometimes and tell me that she loves me. Now, I wouldn't say anything in return, so she said to me, 'Stop being such an Australian and say it back some day.' She thinks Australians don't show emotions, don't tell people how we think and we are all bland people. I think I'm pretty good at telling my family that I love them. But I can't tell people that I love them if I don't. Australians are definitely different to Canadians and I don't think we're huggy people like them. I hate the way all the people at Montreux want to hug all the time.

Sunday, 23 March 1997

Today is Jordan's birthday and I didn't call him. I had so many other things going on in my mind that I didn't realise it was his birthday until tonight.

Let's see, what did I do today? I woke up in a bad mood which got worse as the minutes passed by.

I HATE MONTREUX mainly because they tell me I have to go out and eat every single day. Now they make me go out to eat protein – chicken souvlaki with yoghurt sauce on it which is so scary for me to eat. My workers told me that if I refused to eat it, I'd have to eat three meals out instead of two meals. If I don't eat the chicken souvlaki in 20 minutes, they'll make me eat a beef one instead and I don't eat beef FULL STOP! The people here are so cruel.

I'm not allowed to cry so I just sit in silence a lot. I'm not allowed to be:

Mean

Unpleasant

Quiet
Sad
Unhappy
Cry
Angry
Yell
Scream
Hurt myself
Refuse anything
Run away.

So that pretty well allows me to be emotionless, huh?

Ever since Peggy returned from Hawaii my life has been unbearable. It's OK for her, she doesn't have to feel and deal with the pain everyday like I do. She says I have no manners but I don't know about that. Peggy says she'll help me through this but she isn't helping at all. Right now she's very unwell with pneumonia so she can't help me at all. I feel sorry for her even though I don't like her much right now.

I'm holding so much inside. I'm hurting so badly inside. I'm trying to make it easier on everyone else around me. I'm so afraid, scared and alone.

Just before I finish up I thought I'd do a brief recap of the week. I went out to eat everyday, twice a day on two days. I painted, went for a few walks, played some pool, the piano and on the computer. I spoke to my parents a couple of times. I now call them on Fridays instead of Saturday – Peggy's orders! It was Mum's birthday last week and I was so sorry I missed it but it sounded as if she had a nice day. I miss my family terribly. My heart aches for them.

**

Contact with my family was restricted while I was 'on-care', when I had care workers with me 24 hours a day, every day, and to a large degree later while I was 'off-care', when I didn't have a worker with me at all. This happened because the staff at Montreux had a philosophy that the patients needed to focus on themselves instead of always wanting to care for, and worry about, everyone else, including their family. This restriction applied to phone calls, faxes, family visits, mail, email – all forms of contact. It was done with the patients needs and care in mind but it was very hard on my family and me.

Thursday, 27 March 1997

I was actually in an all right kind of mood when I woke up so I went for a walk down to the beach where it was freezing. When I got back I was weighed and then I had to go out and eat yoghurt at a restaurant. Later, much to my disgust, I had to go out to eat again. This time I had to go to a Greek restaurant to eat a chicken souvlaki cooked in oil and butter! It's so incredibly scary for me. I'm getting bigger and bigger as the days go by.

I have this worker here with me tonight who I just hate. I don't feel safe with her. The only thing she does is make my food and tell me she's going to page Peggy if I do anything wrong. Real nice, ha? So I didn't speak all night and I don't intend on speaking to any- one here ever again. We'll see how long that lasts – probably two or three days.

Friday, 28 March 1997

My stomach really hurts right now. It's Easter this weekend. I think it's so commercialised and quite sad that some people don't even think about the real meaning of Easter.

I'm feeling really angry right now. I hate myself for letting myself go out to eat today. I just want to be alone now.

Peggy told me I can't leave here until I'm well. That could be a really long time and I feel really sorry for everyone who has to put up with me – especially Peggy. I'm so angry with her but I'm angrier with myself for letting it come to this. I feel like I've been punished for doing something really bad, maybe for just being me. Who knows? Anyhow, today was utterly horrible and I want it to be over. I feel like I'm going to burst into tears but I know that I can't. I'm holding so much in. I feel like punching and kicking the walls and yelling and screaming. Oh well.

Sunday, 13 April 1997

HELLO. WELL, HERE I AM ONCE AGAIN WRITING IN HERE. I AM MEGA ANGRY TONIGHT. I MEAN MEGA. I HAD A PRETTY TOUGH DAY. A LONG, LONG DAY. I HAD TO GO OUT TO EAT TWICE TODAY, WHICH WAS HARD FOR ME TO DO. IT'S JUST NOT RIGHT. I'M SO AFRAID OF GAINING WEIGHT. MY BODY DOES NOT KNOW WHAT TO DO WITH ALL THIS EXTRA FOOD. I THINK I'M SCARING IT A LOT.

I DON'T THINK THAT PEGGY AND HER PEOPLE REALISE THE SIDE EFFECTS OF MAKING ME EAT OUT.

Wednesday, 23 April 1997

I hate it here! I'm trapped and I'm stuck in my own world. I hate who I am and what I'm doing. I want to be good, I want to be kind, I want to be gentle and I want to be better. I'm sorry for swearing. I don't belong in this clinic because I don't fit in.

EVERYTHING I DO IS UNSAFE. EVERYTHING I SAY IS BAD. I GET INTO TROUBLE FOR BEING NEGATIVE. PLEASE PROTECT ME FROM MY MONSTER. PLEASE KEEP MY FAMILY AND ME SAFE.

I'M GOING TO PUT ON WEIGHT FROM EATING AND I DON'T WANT TO! I'M AFRAID OF MYSELF. I'M AFRAID OF MY WORKERS. I'M SO AFRAID OF THE FOOD AND THE CONSEQUENCES IN MY MIND! I'M SCARED OF THE WORLD.

Thursday, 1 May 1997

So May has come around which means it's been a year since I left Melbourne and a year since I've had the tube in my nose! I would hate to have that thing in my nose ever again. It's hard to imagine it being there! Oh, hang on a minute. I can imagine it.

So anyway I miss my family. The warmer weather here makes me feel homesick! I had my first tennis lesson the other day! My teacher's name is Rosemary and she must be about 64 years old I reckon. Old or not, she's so nice. I have private lessons with her so I don't have to worry about other people judging me! I was really sore after playing and my muscles are still hurting! Especially in my forearms! I'm getting old.

Friday, 9 May 1997

I'm still playing the piano. I don't want to continue but Peggy won't let me quit! I think it's boring not to mention I'm really bad! But I'll keep playing! It's quite funny because my teacher thinks I can read music but I can't. Got her fooled, I just play by ear.

Saturday, 17 May 1997

Hi! It's me! Imagine that, Bronte writing in her diary. I've been here for a year and 17 days. One year and 17 days too long, if you ask me. I know how much my parents want me to be here. I know in my heart that I need to be here and that I need people with me but it hurts so much and it is so hard to do the things that they want me to do, so incredibly hard!

Eating is still a really hard thing for me to do. It seems really unnatural and so wrong – especially eating out! I've been eating out for nearly three months now, day in and day out, and it's still just so incredibly hard. I can't see past the things I think and feel right now. Someone will tell me something and I'll think they're lying and that everything they say is really the opposite of how it is. Not to mention how huge and disgusting I look now! I'm absolutely MASSIVE and I can't stand it! I hate my personality and the way I look, especially my weight. I wish there were some way I could lose weight without my workers knowing.

Monday, 19 May 1997

I ate out again twice today and it wasn't nice. It's still really hard for me. I feel really guilty after I eat and the voice in my head won't allow me to converse with anyone but myself. I just have to isolate myself to justify my actions.

I hate my body right now. I feel like a huge, ugly, fat PIG! I feel like I'm a walking blob of fat. It's kind of like how anorexia feels inside. It's like a nasty, evil and vindictive monster that won't go away – no matter what you do! I wouldn't wish it upon my worst enemy! No way. I may be mean and cruel – but I'm not that mean.

Tuesday, 20 May 1997

I'm feeling a lot of guilt lately for what I've put my family through. They didn't deserve what I did to them back home and I'm so sorry for being the way I am. But I never wanted it to be like this. I never thought I would have to go to a strange place in Canada and leave my family for such a long length of time. I'm so angry! I just want to kick and scream and cry. I hate what my workers are making me do! It's sickening. I know they're just trying to help me get rid of this anorexia but what they think is helping, in fact, isn't help at all. It's just anger, frustration and pain all rolled up into a ball and thrown at YOU. Some help, ha!

Peggy says I have no reason to be angry and that I should thank her. I don't know why I can't do that. Probably because I'm selfish. I feel bad and sorry for her and everyone else here who has to put up with me while I waste their time, space and money.

Thursday, 5 June 1997

Here's a poem that sums up how I feel at the moment. Writing poetry is an escape from anorexia for a while.

The shadow surrounds you,
Slowly enfolding you,
Into its arms.
Crushing your being and mind,
Each notion and thought,
Until it was you.
Giving you the gift of knowing,
The sense of something, what you are, do and need.
THIS IS ME,
ME THE SHADOW.
The door is closed and locked for good!
Locked in the prison of the shadow.
Once trapped, strangled with fear,
There is no escaping to freedom,
No escaping living life the way it is.
If only I could run from my own mind,
Maybe then I could be free,
Then I wouldn't want to cry.
Being stalked, every move made watched and judged
    upon, assessed and being made justifiable.
Paying for things that make me feel bad!
To see the Sunshine without the cloud would be a nice
    thing to do one day!

Wednesday, 18 June 1997

I feel like my body is turning into a huge balloon. It's
getting bigger and is going to keep getting bigger until
I leave here and then I can lose all the weight.

I'm so scared of change – every thing has to be the
same. How could I let myself be like this? I'm so afraid
of food. I shouldn't be going out anywhere at all to
eat. My workers are trying to make me more scared.

Everyone hates me but I don't blame them. I'm a very boring person. I feel guilty because I'm not better yet. I came to a place to get better and it didn't work. I failed yet again. I failed because I got sick. I always fail.

I'm being strangled by this anorexia – this thing that has become me. Who am I anyway? Why am I so stubborn? Why can't I be helped? Because I'm selfish? Because I'm weak and ungrateful and because people hate Bronte? You have no place in the world, Bronte. Bronte is nothing. Bronte shouldn't eat and will put on weight from eating anything at all.

Why can't people just leave me to do what I want to do? Why won't they tell me the truth? I'm going crazy inside my brain. I can't deal with this. I'm afraid of my own mind – of having a thought and a consequence for every action I make. Everything is my fault. I'm really tired.

I'm surrounded by a huge big black shadow that is strangling me.

I want to cry.

I want to run away forever.

I want to go home.

I want my Dad to hug me.

I am so afraid. Help me.

I'm scared,

I'm scared I wrote this.

In the spring of 1997 I moved to a house that was like a campus of Montreux. It was a 15-minute walk from the Mansion towards the beach. It was another big house but far less grand than the others I'd lived in. It was a house where patients who were off-care and further along in the recovery program lived. I was not off-care and I certainly wasn't near that stage in my program. The hope was that the positive approach to life of the other patients would inspire me.

Richmond House, as I would come to know it, was weatherbeaten and rickety with a genuine falling down look about it. It wasn't that old, just neglected. It wore a tatty overcoat of pale grey shingles and weatherboards while a slate roof sat on top like a crumpled old hat on some hobo's head. Inside, I noticed the eclecticism of the whole house from the rose-coloured carpet to a brick fireplace doubling as a room divider, to the walls covered in sickly green paint.

The house was fragmented into parts yet it was still quite open. It had a communal kitchen, a bathroom, a living and dining room and four bedrooms. My room was at the very front of the house with two windows facing the quiet street. My walls were mint green, which took my breath away, but it wasn't until I looked down at the sad brown shag pile carpet that I was truly shocked. This room was in serious need of a paint job and I decided to repaint the walls to a fresh hue of yellow so that the shag carpet wouldn't seem so bad. At first the whole communal living thing freaked me out but it was actually a huge plus as it forced me to interact with the other Montreux residents for the first time.

The house was full of girls except for the one token male, Charlie. How he put up with the complete 'girlieness' of the place is beyond me. The bathroom window wouldn't stay open and was propped up with boxes of sanitary products. It was here at Richmond House that

I got to know Charlie, and it was here that I formed my friendship with Kornelia, an eccentric German who brightened every one of my days at that house – she will be a friend forever.

Kornelia was twenty-three when I met her and wasn't one for birthdays. She would climb out of windows at all hours of the morning to avoid a rendition of *Happy Birthday* from me. Kornelia couldn't escape for long though. At some point she would have to come home and I would sing it to her when she came back. Kornelia was very tall and very blonde. She had wonderful blue eyes and her complexion was like fine porcelain. She was a gentle soul and a tower of strength for me. Her quirkiness and humour got me through many hard days.

It was in Richmond House, and with friends like Charlie and Kornelia, that I began to want to recover for me. I began to slowly move forward. I still fought change. I fought trying new food and going out to eat. A lot of pain was still to come.

Friday, 20 June 1997

Dear Mum,

Right now I'm painting my room because I've moved house yet again. I now live at Richmond House, which is a 5-minute drive from the Mansion. Peggy calls Richmond the happy house. There are six other people who live in the house with me and they're all really nice, fun people to be around. There's even a dog that lives at the house, a Doberman, and her name is Madison.

Anyway, I moved down here about four days ago. I have my own room but when I moved in it was a light green colour that reminded me of a hospital. I decided to paint it a light creamy yellow colour called Italian Straw. I'm painting the trim a midnight blue. It's a lot of work; I'll send you a photo when I finish it.

So anyway Mum, I love you and here's a really big hug on paper from me. Please take good care of your-self. Give Dad a kiss for me, eh! Oh, and send my love to Sam, Jordan, James and the hounds.

Thinking of you always.

Your one and only,

Bronte

I spent my mornings at Richmond House getting ready and preparing food for the day. My worker and I would walk to the Mansion to paint with Irma, visit Noah, check the mail and emails and then go to an Educational Program for a few hours in the afternoon. Three times a week I would have a counselling session at the Fort Street office, which was a 10-minute walk towards the city from the Mansion. This was another Montreux offshoot, but was only used from 9 to 5 as an office. By the time I got back to the Richmond House my evening worker would greet me and Kornelia would be home from her daily activities.

Nights would be spent watching *Absolutely Fabulous* on television or creating some crazy piece of poetry or planning our next surprise birthday party for a house-mate. If Charlie was around he would organise some bizarre outing for us all. He founded the Richmond House Tennis Club and we all became instant members even if we couldn't, or didn't want to, play tennis.

We would also watch the *Austin Powers* films in an old aeroplane hangar that we temporarily transformed into a cinema with over-stuffed vintage couches and chairs. Charlie would try to get us to dress up in 1960s clothes he found at a second-hand shop. The outfits were mostly tight, green and sleazy which was perfect for the occasion. I wouldn't wear any piece of second-hand clothing with my germ phobia so I went as myself. It was one of the many hilarious nights we had. But this created another problem for me – having fun made me feel guilty.

One sunny morning, right on cue for my second snack, I got my yoghurt and fruit from the fridge and began pouring it into my bowl. I hadn't measured it out. Instantly, I freaked out and tried to pour the yoghurt back into the measuring mug. I was in tears but my workers saw an opportunity for a major breakthrough in my recovery. From now on, they told me, I wasn't allowed to measure my food.

The Richmond House crew became family to me and we did just about everything together. Watching these people embrace who they were and life was incredible to me. It made me excited that perhaps recovery was possible. Yet I was also terrified that I was so different and the exception to the rule, that I would never be able to do what they could or be a part of their world. This never stopped them involving me and continuously pushing me to challenge my boundaries. I became an integral part of this house and its dynamics. We were all going through a painful process of recovery from an eating disorder. We cried together and we laughed together.

Life was never dull at Richmond House. I would hear a knock on my door at 10 p.m. and Charlie would announce there was a serious game of Twister happening in the lounge room and that I had to join in. On Wednesday nights I would go to pottery classes. Without fail, I would be picked up after class in the clinic's Nissan van greeted by half the household. We would open the sunroof, crank up the CD player and sing our hearts out all the way home. I would then head off for bed to find Charlie and Kornelia hanging out in my room waiting for my worker to leave so we could have a deep and meaningful conversation. Charlie taught me the art of soccer and how to celebrate a goal while Kornelia taught me the meaning of being accepted for who I truly am, a gift I will never forget.

Thursday, 17 July 1997

Dear Dad,

I've been feeling really, really homesick lately. I got out the photos of home and looked at them all. I have a corkboard hanging on the wall at the end of my bed. I have lots of pictures of you, Mum, Jordan, James, Sam, [and the dogs] Muffin and Mac. I have one photo of Nanny and Poppa.

Life is tough, isn't it? Being here is without doubt the hardest thing I've ever had to do in my life. Do you know it's been 15 months, so a year and a bit, since I had the tube in my nose? I still remember it so well. I get phantom pains sometimes and my nose bleeds quite a bit but it's all right. I want you to know that as tough as it is, I'm not giving up. I'm not going to quit. I'm trying really hard, even though I feel horrible.

Bronte

Tuesday, 22 July 1997

I've been told that I have to go to breakfast tomorrow. I really don't want to face breakfast but I will try. At least Kornelia will be there which should make the whole experience a little less torturous, I hope.

One Sunday night the phone rang. It was Peggy inviting the Richmond House mob out to dinner. It would be the first time I had ever eaten out with anyone other than my workers and the first time eating out in a group. This time it wasn't just about the fear of the food, it was also a fear of socialising. After dinner, my roommates took me to the beach, a 10 minute walk down the road to help me get my mind off the meal. It was summer and warm but darkness was beginning to surround us as we set off. All six residents of Richmond House marched in silence, hand-in-hand spread across the road. It must have been a weird sight. There was an unspoken strength within each of us that night. We fought together like soldiers in a war, brothers in arms.

By mid-1997 a 'dining-out' group was formed with the aim of going out for breakfast and dinner. I hated going. Imagine, one counsellor and nine anorexia and bulimia sufferers freaking out at the prospect of ordering off the menu and then trying to eat the food. The rule was that we all had to sit at the table until everyone had finished. This wouldn't have been so bad if it weren't for the same patients taking at least two hours to eat every meal. It made the experience so much more painful for the rest of us as we waited for the last person to finish. Every time I got home from one of these 'dining-out' experiences I would be completely panic-stricken and want to exercise excessively or starve myself for the rest of the day. My workers would never allow me to follow through on these thoughts, which would annoy me no end.

A light-bulb must have gone off in a counsellor's head and after three months of torturous 'dining-out' dates the group was scrapped, but my eating out days were far from over. They were just beginning. I now started going out for lunch and I was told that I had to try different food. Whenever I was faced with a new food challenge I longed for that little muffin back at the old musty tea-house. How easy that seemed compared to what was now before me. I would go with little resistance but I would struggle to eat my next snack because I felt I had eaten too much at lunch. I would feel so full that I thought I would burst. I would feel full for hours, even days, after I had eaten something I considered to be 'scary' food – which was anything except fish and vegetables.

I now know that to feel full so long after eating a meal is impossible but that was my reality back then. Mind over matter. It wasn't until I tried these foods over and over again and continued eating my meal plan at the clinic, and not compensating, that I began to discover that nothing happened to my body when I ate.

Friday, 15 August 1997

Angry
Frustrated
Hopeless
Never-ending pain and fear
Hatred
Worthlessness
Trapped
Scared and very alone
Locked in my own world

I wish I was alone in a place where no one else existed. No one could pretend to care and no one could hurt me. 'He' couldn't hurt me because we would be one once more. No one could touch us, no one could trap us. No fears would exist in our world, for there would be no one to care about or hurt. No possessions, no people. No enemies except myself. But I wish I was free. Never to be trapped. Never to be scared, afraid or alone.

I'm a bad person and everyone believes and thinks that. That's why Mum and Dad sent me to a place where I would get yelled at for being so bad and selfish. I don't deserve a place in this world. I don't deserve a loving family. I don't deserve happiness and freedom. I wouldn't be missed. Maybe it's best if I disappear.

Saturday, 30 August 1997

The camera crew from Channel Nine are arriving tomorrow. My Mum is coming with them so at least that's a positive. Mum says Ray Martin isn't coming though as he's going to London to cover the death of Princess Diana. I don't want anyone to come but they're on their way. Not much I can do about it. A man called Rob Penfold is coming instead of Ray. I'm really scared to talk to him because I don't know him from a bar of soap. Mum has told me he's really nice so that makes me feel a little better.

When I arrived in Canada I thought, thankfully, that was the end of my media career. How wrong I was. Again, I don't remember ever saying, 'Sure, why don't you come and film me going through hell trying to recover.' But somehow it just seemed to happen again. The media and Montreux didn't mix well for me and it was here that a number of conflicts arose. During my time in Canada I began to wish that I'd never become involved with any media and I became quite angry when Channel Nine wanted to film me. Battling anorexia day in and day out was exhausting enough without having to let an entire nation watch me do it.

At the time I arrived in 1996, Montreux was attracting a lot of media attention from around the world wanting to see what the controversial clinic was up to. There was no great hidden secret, really. It's just that anorexia makes good television, sells magazines and is therefore always on the media radar screens. The clinic staff insisted I speak with these television crews and let them see what my anorexia was like. I felt obligated and guilty if I didn't do it. So not only did I have the media from home but now I had to face the media from Europe and North America as well.

The first visit from A Current Affair in Canada was in late August of 1997 after I had been at the clinic for eighteen months. The idea freaked me out completely. I was terribly afraid that I wasn't well enough for people from the 'outside world' to see me and that everyone who would watch the show would see the clinic and me as failures. From this fear came the idea that I had to pretend to be 'better' so as to make everyone happy. That's not to say I wasn't getting better. Don't get me wrong. I was getting better but the whole process was taking so long. I began to self-edit what I told the cameras.

Later on Mum told me a funny story about the planning

of this visit by Channel Nine. She said she had been working closely with Ray's producer, Steve Bibb, to organise the
filming in Canada. Towards the end of their planning, and
just before their departure, Mum told Steve to enjoy the trip
and hopefully nothing major would happen. When asked
what she meant, Mum pointed out that the Port Arthur
massacre happened on the day they took me to Canada on
28 April 1996. Steve reassured Mum that all would be fine
and nothing would stop them from seeing me in Canada.
Nobody expected that fatal accident in a Paris tunnel.
Mum was spookily right again.

Monday, 8 September 1997

*I feel like everyone hates me because I'm stupid. I feel
fat. Kirsten – my counsellor – doesn't like me. She
thinks I'm a loser. I know she likes everyone else more
than me. That goes for everyone here. I can't even say
what I think and feel because no one really wants to
hear what I have to say. I feel hopeless like there's no
end to anorexia and all the fears I live with. I feel like
a failure.*

Tuesday, 9 September 1997

*I think the constant handwashing thing is never going
to change, nor my fear of food, nor my fear of disease.
And I do NOT want to think these horrible, awful
thoughts any more. I don't want to be afraid of
getting up and living every single day of my life.*

*I feel like I'm not as good as other people. I'm much
more boring and annoying. I feel like I can't learn so I'll
never get past this anorexia. My family probably don't
like me after all I've put them through. I'm definitely*

a failure compared to the others. Sam, Jordan, James,
Mum and Dad are all such wonderful people. They
are all smart. I'm not.

My story ran on *A Current Affair* on the night of
9 September 1997, right across Australia. I've never seen
the story, and never want to see it. I just don't like looking at myself on television. My parents received hundreds
of letters from viewers who were glad to find out how
I was doing in Canada. Amazingly, some people even sent
money to my parents.

9/9/97
Dear Cullis Family,
    I was touched by your daughter's story and her struggles
with anorexia. She is truly a girl who has turned her life around.
I look forward to maybe reading her book if she ever writes one
or seeing her artistic talent displayed, only time will tell.
    Thank you for your devotion and care, and concern and love
and especially the lengths you have gone through to provide
Bronte with a fighting chance.
    My heart goes out to you as a family and may God bless you.
May this cheque and many more like it help to ease the load.
With love and concern
Sandy

10/9/97
Dear Mr and Mrs Cullis,
    Not being a regular watcher of television I had not seen
your story before last night. What I saw has moved me to write
to you and send you some money to help in some small way.
    It was the two of you, as parents, who've inspired me to do this.
Both of you are willing to give everything for your daughter and yet
it is not a sacrifice but what you do because you are good parents.

Your actions remind me of my relationship with my parents. All my life I have known, and been told by words and actions that if I need help all I have to do is ask and I will have it. I know if I was in your daughter's situation my parents would do as you have done.

Your daughter is courageous, and I'm sure she will become an exceptional adult with a lot to give back to society, not just because of the disease she is fighting, but because with two parents like you as role models she is learning the true meaning of unconditional love.

Your children are very lucky to have parents like you.
Kind regards,
JJ

12.9.97
To Bronty [sic] and Mr and Mrs Cullis,
I wish I had more to help and hope many people are doing like-wise. People power will over-come this and bless you for the fight. You see I do know. I'm 38 now and relatively okay but I remember.

Bless you
Vivien

11-9-97
Bronte,
I'm 44, married, two kids – you're a battler – keep fighting, kiddo – you can do it! We're proud of you!
Love DB

Dear Bronte's Family,
My heart went out to you the other night on A Current Affair. My niece 15yrs has just gone into the North Shore clinic for anorexia. One day's progress seems to take about 1 month if we are lucky.

I wish I could do more for you.

I look forward [to] hearing more about Bronte's progress. After seeing Bronte we now know that there is light at the end of that very long tunnel, we might not be able to see it now, but we will one day.

All my Love
Penny

12th September 1997
Mr and Mrs Cullin [sic],

Please accept this cheque on behalf of the residents of —— House Youth Refuge who have decided to donate their combined rent for a week.

This money is normally banked for their use for luxury items such as take-away, movies, videos, etc.

After hearing your story on A Current Affair, the residents made a joint decision to help Bronte.

I think the fact that she has such wonderful and supportive parents touched the hearts of so many people and made them want to ensure Bronte's continued success.

Wishing you and Bronte a wonderful future,
Administrator on behalf of residents.

Monday, 22 September 1997

My stomach feels really, really huge. I'm frightened because I ate toast with jam and peanut butter. I can't stop thinking about my breakfast this morning. I know I'm gaining weight from it. I shouldn't have gone out so much today. I feel selfish and very ugly. I'm worrying about so many things.

I feel really bad for not calling my family today. I just ran out of time.

Tuesday, 30 September 1997

I feel very, very guilty about the pizza I ate today. I feel like it's more than I usually eat for protein. I'm so angry that I have to eat this stuff. My stomach hurt all night because of the pizza. There was so much cheese and sauce and oil on it. Peggy wouldn't let me go for a walk to burn off the fat, which upsets me no end. I can't sit still.

My stomach feels humongous. I can't stand it right now. It's driving me mad. I'm fat, ugly and annoying. I'm selfish and worthless.

My needs are less than others yet I feel as if I demand so much more. I'm less important than anyone else in the world. I feel guilty for speaking with people.

Charlie packed up to go home in September of 1997, leaving Kornelia and me devastated. He had really grown into a man, an adorable one at that. The house just wasn't the same without him. It seemed to have lost its sparkle. Not long after that Kornelia moved into an apartment in the city.

Charlie sent postcards of his adventures and the world outside Montreux. His words inspired me to want life. Kornelia's move out on her own pushed me that little bit further. I felt left behind and I wanted to know what it was like to be in their shoes out there living life.

Friday, 17 October 1997

I remember being young and afraid of so many things. I've never really lived, never experienced anything but my own world. My voice tells me to jump high, jump low, round about, skip, hop, spit, run, walk, walk faster, ride, do this, do that, do this, do that. Not knowing which way to turn because there's always something there that scares me. Thinking about every consequence of every action I make every day of my life. Having to follow routines and rituals. I'm so afraid. I think I'll live like this forever – being petrified of food, running, hiding and living my life in fear. I can't describe the pain. It's so black. I can't see past the blackness right now.

Right now? Right now I'm doing things that are wrong. I feel guilty and bad. Maybe some people never get better; maybe some people aren't worth the effort of trying to help. I feel isolated from everyone, totally alone. I try to distract my thoughts but it doesn't always work. I go deeper inside. Not talking is a way I deal with pain, anger and frustration. I figure if I'm going to get into trouble for speaking up, I just won't do it any more. That way everyone will think I'm just fine. They'll leave me alone and I can go home and lose as much weight as I want to. But then I would upset my family and I don't want to do that. Maybe I will just have to go and live on my own.

Sunday, 19 October 1997

My family think I don't like them yet I love them more than anyone else! I'm just a mean, selfish, fat, disgusting, ugly person who only thinks of herself.

I'm so afraid of eating and I don't know if I can do it any more. I can't deal with the repercussions eating has on my body. I was fat in hospital back home but

I've become even fatter here. I feel like I'm going crazy inside.

I wish I could sit down with someone to tell them of the fears that control my life. You can't expect me to come to a place and in a year and a half just try to change my lifelong fears. NO! Everyone thinks I'm just a big pretender. Well, newsflash, I'm not pretending. There's so much going on in my mind that I just wouldn't tell anyone. As I wrote before, if I don't say anything they'll think I'm fine and therefore ship me home.

This is my whole life; I can't change. And just because some person – who's supposed to know anorexia inside and out – tells you that it's going to go away doesn't mean it will happen.

Peggy says people here have shown me that what I think, or what anorexia thinks, is wrong. Well, if that's true then why do I still think the same things? I can't believe anyone. I don't know who to trust.

I want to go home. I miss my family. I miss my bed. I should be with my family in Australia. I don't belong here. I go to bed most nights and cry myself to sleep. Cry in fear and of loneliness (I know Peggy would tell me I'm not lonely because I always have someone beside me). Well, let me say that even though there are people there, sometimes they may as well not be.

Anyway I've really just been writing this worthless piece of rubbish and I can't decide whether to throw it away or keep it. I've probably just wasted a tree.

Friday, 5 December 1997

I feel extremely overwhelmed today because of all the different foods I've been eating. My stomach feels enormous and I know it's because of the two pancakes with butter and syrup I ate for breakfast.

I had a change in my protein this afternoon. It was salmon and it tasted slimy and fatty. I felt guilty eating it because it was different and I don't know how many calories are in salmon!

My worker and I went to a chemist but I didn't want to stay because there were too many people. We also went to a video store but I couldn't touch anything because it's all dirty and 'germy'.

I didn't wash my hands much this morning. The people here at the clinic are trying to confront my rituals, and handwashing is a good one. I had to go to the bathroom but my workers wouldn't let me wash my hands more than once. How hard is that! I was scared that my hands were dirty because I hadn't washed them for so long.

It makes me so mad that I have no control over so many things. My head is killing me at the moment with terrible thoughts. For example, my weight is sky-rocketing out of control and there's nothing I can do about it! My stomach is so ROUND I can't even wear my jeans because they're too tight! Everything is too tight and it's so hard to keep doing all the things the people here ask me to do. I feel like I'm just doing all these crazy things but I don't really know why.

Everyone thinks I should be past the worst of this disease so I'll tell them what I really think! I can't believe how BIG I'm becoming. I can't write any more now because I am getting upset. Help me.

Saturday, 6 December 1997

My stomach is absolutely enormous today. It looks too big and feels SO BIG! I felt like crying many times today. I had to do my laundry but I can't fold the clothes because I think my hands are dirty.

I didn't call my parents yesterday and I feel very mean about that. My head won't allow me to go out or do anything I like.

Everything around me is dirty. The couches in the living room have red marks on them, which I think is blood and I don't want to sit on them. If I do sit on them I'll have to wash my clothes immediately.

My head kept telling me to wash my hands after I touched anything today. The only time I'm allowed to wash my hands is when I use the bathroom. If my workers caught me washing my hands any other time they would page Peggy – and I don't want that to happen. I don't feel like getting into trouble from her. I don't like my workers. I find them all very annoying and I wish this day would end.

Peggy and my counsellors were the instigators, or approved, of changes within my program whether it be food, ritualistic behaviour or exercise. On occasions Kirsten would change my meal plan by introducing new food to challenge me, such as the time I had to eat pita bread and hummus. I would always freak out at any change. Any change was too much change. Change would happen whether I liked it or not. So I would deal with it, learn from it and just get comfortable with it until another change was made.

Body image was always a concern for me throughout my treatment at Montreux. It became more acute as I confronted food challenges. Any time a change was made with my food, or a 'scary' food was introduced to my meal plan, it would terrify me. By this stage I was comfortable eating fish as one of my protein snacks for my daily meal plan. The next challenge was to replace the fish with a chicken meal. This was a huge hurdle as chicken was on my list of 'scary' foods. My idea of what I looked like and what was happening to me would overwhelm me and totally cloud any reality. The more pressure my anorexia was under the more I thought my body was expanding.

Sunday, 7 December 1997

Today my stomach is huge because of the peanut butter, jam and bread I ate. Peggy told me that I'm not gaining weight but I think, feel and see that I am. I don't see how someone can sit there and tell me that peanut butter isn't going to put weight on me. Sure!

My stomach is so round and my legs are so wide that when I sit down they look even more enormous. I think I'm stashing all the excess weight and fat on my body and there's nothing I can do about it! I can actually grab chunks of my stomach and when I bend over it rolls and rolls with fat.

We were sitting watching television this morning and a story came on about that disease that I'm really scared of. My head told me that I'll get that blood disease if I gain more weight or don't wash my hands more often.

I'm sitting on my floor and now I think that I can't sit on my bed because I'll make it dirty. When I was putting my clothes away I found a Band-Aid in the bottom of my laundry basket. It was my Band-Aid but I still think it made my clothes dirty.

No one else seems to put on weight from eating the kind of food that I eat, only me. No one sees what I see. I never walk enough because I'm too lazy. I need to walk more, or do some other form of exercise, especially eating the kinds of food that I eat.

I'm trying to get better but I don't feel like I'm getting anywhere. I feel greedy, guilty and bad for eating the things I do. I'm a failure for thinking the things I do.

Monday, 8 December 1997

I went out for breakfast this morning and ate muesli.

I feel like I have no control over my food or weight. It drives me crazy. I hate my stomach. I feel so huge and I see myself putting on more and more weight and nobody sees what I'm saying. It makes me so angry.

My fingers have cuts on them which are scaring me. I keep putting Band-Aids on them but they keep falling off. I feel so guilty about eating new food. I feel guilty about going out to breakfast as well. I should just sit on my bed to eat. I feel like I try so hard yet I don't get anywhere.

Wednesday, 10 December 1997

I ate three pancakes for breakfast this morning. My stomach still feels like it's going to explode. The more

I stuff into my stomach the BIGGER and BIGGER it gets. I also had to eat my Nutribar tonight and have different veggies. I feel so guilty for eating different things. I think I should just stay in my room, not speak and not do anything or go anywhere. I think everyone at the clinic dislikes me and they think I'm fine and can do everything by myself.

I'm so fat and so annoying. I feel alone and lost. No one listens to me. No one wants to listen to me. I'm just a mean fat PIG!

I spoke to Dad today and he sounded upset. Please don't be upset, Dad.

Thursday, 11 December 1997

I decided to have a shower before breakfast today. I thought that way my stomach wouldn't look so bad, so bloated. But I was wrong. My stomach was so big and I hadn't even eaten yet. I'm just getting bigger all the time. This makes me mad.

Friday, 12 December 1997

I think all my food is full of sugar which will make me fat. No one listens when I tell them how BIG I've become. Why don't they listen to me? I must be twice the size of anyone else at the clinic.

I have to wash my hands because they're always dirty. Everything I touch makes them dirty. I get angry with my workers for telling me what to do all the time. Give me a break!

I don't want to keep eating different things. I can't even wear clothes that touch my waist. I'm only usually comfortable in overalls and today I'm not even *comfortable in those! They feel tight – especially around my stomach and legs.*

I'm afraid to write in this diary and to tell people what I really think in my head. They will tell me that I shouldn't have these issues, just like Peggy did tonight. Who's right – my head or the workers? I feel like such a loser.

I think no one likes me or even wants to bother with me. I shouldn't speak to anyone because they probably don't want to listen to me anyway. I'm not a very exciting person to talk to or be around. That's probably why Mary, Peggy and Nicole don't want to talk to me any more.

Mary was a patient living in St Charles at Montreux when I arrived. She was in her late teens, tall, had long straight ochre-coloured hair and beautiful big blue eyes. She was from England and had the most perfect accent. I warmed to Mary as soon as we met. I got to know her quite well and soon discovered that our illnesses were very similar in the way we thought and acted. Mary was a strength and constant motivation for me. It was encouraging to watch others recover around me and see that 'life beyond anorexia' was possible. Mary eventually went back to England.

Wednesday, 17 December 1997

I went to the corner store tonight. The guy serving me had open cuts on his hands and I think there's blood on the things I bought. Now I don't want to use them because I think I'll get that bad disease.

My jacket got really dirty today because I was using

*it to touch the door handles at the shopping centre
and bank. Now I have to wash it. My bankcard is dirty
too from that guy touching it at the corner store.*

*I had to go out for breakfast this morning and
Justin my worker tried to make me eat the hot cereal
with brown sugar. I just can't eat that because I'm
so afraid sugar will put on weight. I had the muesli
instead and that's also really frightening because it has
so many calories in it.*

*Tonight I had to eat the alternative snack of pretzel
with jam and cream cheese. I feel guilty for eating it
and my stomach feels and looks enormous. I feel like
my body weight is way out of control. It scares me.*

Thursday, 18 December 1997

I feel scared.

I feel greedy.

I feel selfish.

*My hands were dirty when I had to go to the bath-
room.*

I'm greedy because I make my food.

*I know, feel and see that I'm gaining weight from what
I eat. I'm frightened.*

Friday, 19 December 1997

*I'm scared of lots of things right now. I just finished
eating my last muffin snack for the day and my stomach looks enormous. I feel so sad and angry about it.
Other people don't gain weight from eating, but I do.*

*There was some fresh laundry on my bed and
I couldn't put it away until I'd washed my hands
otherwise I would have made my clothes dirty.*

Shar my worker helped me arrange the Christmas cards people have sent me. I feel bad looking at them because I don't know why those people wanted to send me a card. I don't deserve them. I feel like I'll be here forever. Like I'll never be free from this.

I could never wear my clothes twice. Everything had to be washed as soon as I wore it. Nothing could go back in the wardrobe to be worn another day because I was convinced the clothes would be covered in germs that would make me sick with AIDS. So my laundry pile was always ten times higher than it should have been. I never felt clean. To me it seemed germs were over every-thing and so I started showering more. My usual was three and each time I had a shower I had to wear a new set of freshly-washed clothes. It quickly became a real battle as my carers struggled to stop me showering and changing clothes.

Wednesday, 24 December 1997

Mum arrived by herself today from Australia to spend Christmas with me. I love spending time with her. She plans to be here until just after my birthday in January.

Thursday, 25 December 1997

Christmas Day. I should feel happy but instead I feel greedy and guilty because people bought me presents. I shouldn't get anything as I certainly haven't done anything to deserve presents. I shouldn't have sent Christmas cards because who would want anything from me? I didn't buy enough Christmas presents for other people and that makes me feel selfish.

My hands were dirty today and I hardly got a chance to wash them. I had to keep pretending I needed to use the toilet so I could sneak in a hand wash.

I feel I'm a nasty person. My mind is telling me I've got the bad disease (yes, that one!) from all the bad things I do such as not washing my hands enough. I can't sit when I'm wearing my pyjamas because that would make my bed dirty and then I'll have to wash the sheets before I get in again. I'm always making things dirty.

Sunday, 28 December 1997

Yesterday I was walking down the street and there appeared to be blood on the ground. I walked around it but I still think it got on my shoes and now I think my pants and shoes are contaminated.

I feel so alone because I have to do everything myself and no one wants to help me.

I feel guilty about not being with my Mum all the time while she's here visiting me. I feel obliged to entertain her 24 hours a day. I think she doesn't like me. I think she thinks I'm mean. I just want to make her happy. I just want to make everyone else happy. I fear I'll never feel different than this. It's awful. I feel like giving up.

I've been washing my hands a lot more this weekend.

1998

Saturday, 3 January 1998

It's my birthday today. I'm 19. Happy birthday to me. Mum is here. I went out for breakfast today with Kornelia at the beautiful Empress Hotel downtown and ate SO MUCH! I had to eat oatmeal with dried fruit and I had a whole container of brown sugar on it. I know it's going to put so much weight on me. I feel disgusting, fat and ugly. I feel angry with myself for eating food that terrifies me. I put on weight and no one listens to me. We met with Mum after breakfast.

Tuesday, 6 January 1998

I spent too much money buying a ticket to the movies today. I feel greedy and selfish. I still feel guilty because so many people gave me too many Christmas presents. The jacket I wore today was a birthday present from Mum. She told me she bought it after it was returned to the store so I washed it in hot water but I still think it's dirty and that I'll get germs from it. I had to touch some money to pay for CDs I bought and I'm scared I'll get sick from the germs because the money was dirty.

Wednesday, 7 January 1998

I went out for breakfast and ate two extremely large pieces of FRENCH TOAST! I'm so afraid that I'm gaining so MUCH weight. Why is it that no one else can see this except me? Everyone must think I'm the MOST hugest person in this clinic.

My head is really loud and angry with me for going out for breakfast. It's mad because I try to be nice to people when they're mean and make me do things I don't want to do. I don't understand why I have to go out to eat when I see myself gaining weight every time I go out to eat.

I didn't wash my hands enough today. People were touching me after touching a video from the store. I think I got germs from that.

Friday, 9 January 1998

I'm selfish because I've been out too much and I've seen too many movies. I spend too much money and other people spend too much money on me!

Today Shar put the bracelet I got for my birthday in a drawer in my room. I think the drawer has contaminated the bracelet so now I can't wear it. I still won't use the hair gel I bought from the chemist. I think it's dirty because a person serving me in the chemist touched it.

I feel like a failure.

I feel stupid and dumb.

I feel like I'll never get better.

Like I'll never get past my fears.

Saturday, 10 January 1998

My body is so, so disgusting. I revolt even myself. I'll never feel any better than this. No one here cares or wants to listen. Can you blame them? My stomach and legs are absolutely enormous.

I don't do enough exercise. I need to walk more. I feel guilty for so many things that I do in my day and I worry too! I worry a lot about so many things.

I talk too much. No one wants to see me or talk to me. I think my counsellors don't want to listen to me because I'm so repetitive and I'm so dumb.

I think bad things always happen to me but not to anyone else. Everyone else can get well but not me. I'm stupid and selfish. I had to put the gel in my hair yesterday and I'm afraid that I got germs. Shar told me that I had to use the gel so I had no choice.

I think my family doesn't like me because I'm mean, selfish, greedy and fat and that I'm a failure.

Wednesday, 21 January 1998

I feel hopeless because I've been here too long and I'll never change or get fully better. Maybe there is no better.

I had to wash my hands a lot as they're always dirty. The taps are dirty too so now I think every time I wash my hands I make them dirty again. Someone was washing their hands at the kitchen sink after using the bathroom, getting all their germs on the taps. I had to wash my hands this morning before I got my clothes ready because Kornelia had been touching my hands and she had been handling dirty money.

My head still won't let me speak to anyone after I eat.

Tuesday, 27 January 1998

I'm losing control over my food intake. It's all because I'm having a lot of trouble coping with not measuring my yoghurt, fruit and sweet potato and potato. It's really, really frightening. I'm worried my weight is changing so much. I really must be allowed to measure my food. It's not safe to do otherwise. It's not structured, so it's not safe. I know there is always more when I have to do it 'free hand'. I'm angry, so angry about doing it and when Kirsten, my counsellor, told me that I have to go out with her to eat an ice-cream, it made me even madder. I cannot do that! My body will stash the weight. My stomach is enormous. It's HUGE, DISGUSTING. The more I don't measure, the BIGGER I GET.

One of my vitamins was broken but I ate it any way. I'm now scared that maybe someone had tampered with it. What will happen to me?

I think I shouldn't have singing lessons any more because I'm not good at it and I don't think I ever will be.

I'm really ugly and I can say that because today I saw photos of me and I don't want anyone else to see them.

Wednesday, 28 January 1998

Today was really, really, really difficult. Breakfast terrified me. It was a cinnamon and apple bun with walnuts, sugar and icing. It was huge and extremely frightening. Boy, do I feel bad about eating it. I can't believe I ate it.

My hands started bleeding when I was at the shopping mall today because I've been washing them so much. They are so dry and cracked. Everything I touched today was dirty. My head is telling me to wash my hands again.

Thursday, 29 January 1998

I spoke to Mum and Dad today. Dad called and I think I wasn't cheery enough for them. I tried to be happy for them. I don't want them to worry about me but I do worry about them so much. I want them to be safe and happy. My Dad said he wants to go out to eat with me and Mum the next time they visit Canada. This makes me feel like a failure too. I can't even imagine doing that. I just want to hide from everything right now. I don't want to face anything. I feel lost, unsafe, insecure and alone even though there are people around me. I feel controlled by my feelings. I'm angry that I'm so afraid of so many things. I'm angry that I don't believe in myself enough to see that change is possible.

Friday, 30 January 1998

I had a meeting with Peggy that upset me so much. She said she was going to take Shar, my worker, away from me. Shar is the one person I can rely on and I'm expected to battle through on my own! I'm angry and I feel desperate. I feel like this struggle is never ending and that things will never be good for me no matter how hard I try.

**

Shar had become an incredibly knowledgeable care worker after spending eighteen testing months by my side. When a new patient arrived at Montreux in need of a fantastic worker, Shar was the obvious choice. I was angry and sad that she was leaving me even though I knew deep down someone else needed her more than I did.

At this point in my treatment, I really had come as far as I could with Shar. In order to move forward we needed to let go of each other. For me that meant new workers and for Shar it meant new clients.

As my condition was challenged at Montreux my phobia about germs and my obsessive need to wash my hands got worse. One fear replaced another and it appeared to me as if I was never going to get better.

Although the thoughts in my diary entries at this time are negative and seem hopeless, I was getting better. Some days I could see the changes I'd made and how far I'd come. Other days, the really hard days, I just couldn't see my progress. This was because I was constantly working on something such as a fear, an obsession or a ritual. Even though some things were so much better, at the time the immediate challenge before me often clouded my vision of any progress.

Friday, 6 February 1998

I can't sleep. I'm just lying here thinking about a lot of things and worrying. I was so mean to people today. I was swearing and shouting. I'm so frustrated, annoyed and mad. I worry so much about not measuring my food and about eating different food from my regular meal plan.

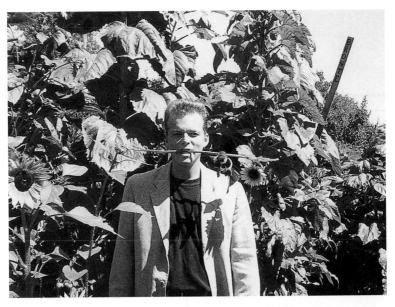

Noah, one of the managers at Montreux, in front of the sunflower garden that I planted.

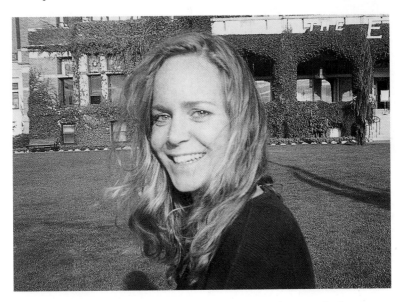

Cindy, one of my care workers and my first team leader, outside the Empress Hotel in downtown Victoria.

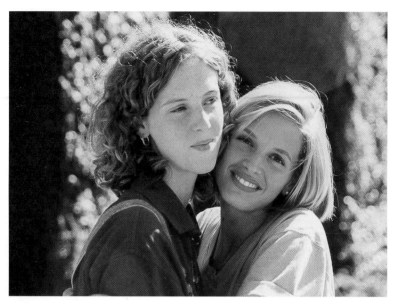

Shar, one of my care workers and later my team leader, and me outside the Empress Hotel in the summer of 1997.

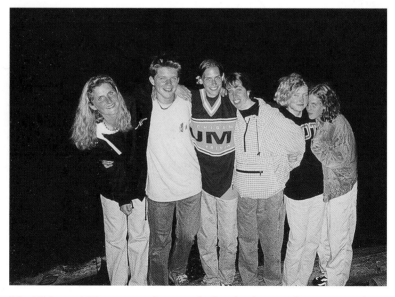

The Richmond House gang down at the beach after our dinner out with Peggy. From left: Charlotte, Charlie, Rachael, Melissa, Kornelia and me.

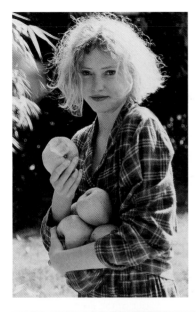

Kornelia on a summer morning at Richmond House.
(Photo: Nicole Claude-Pierre)

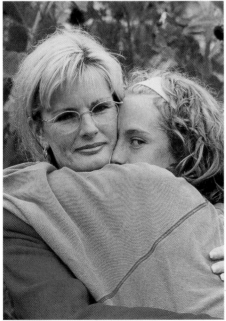

Mum and me in the garden at Montreux during one of her visits in 1997.

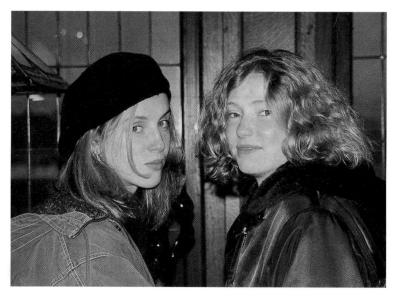

Kornelia and me on my 19th birthday taking a tour of the Empress Hotel.

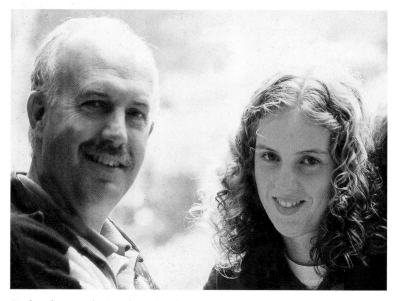

Dad and me at the Butchart Gardens in Victoria in 1998.

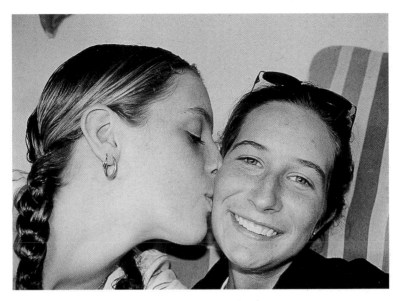

Becca and me hanging out in my suite at St Charles in 1998.

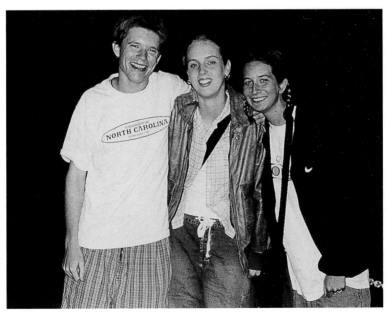

Charlie, me and Becca at the inner harbour during one of Charlie's visits after he'd left Montreux.

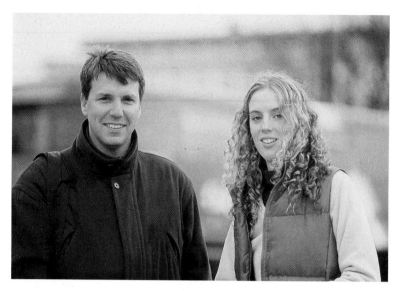

Steve Bibb and me during a week of filming in Victoria, Canada, 1999.

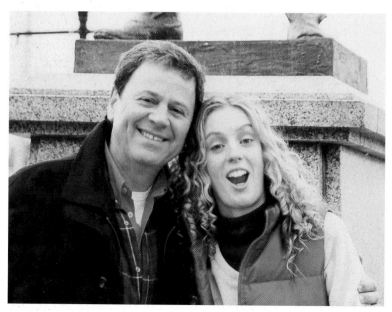

Ray Martin and me standing under a statue of James Cook in Victoria.

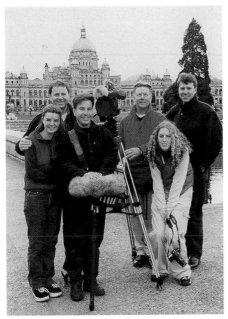

My sister Sam, Ray, Joe, Steff, me and Steve taking a break from filming around inner harbour.

Below: Linda, one of my care workers, and me at the 21st birthday party a few of my friends and workers at Montreux threw for me.

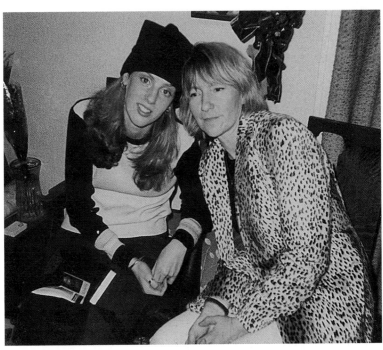

Margie Bashfield, from Channel Nine, and me at my 21st birthday party during a visit home to Melbourne in March 2000.

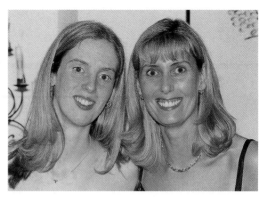

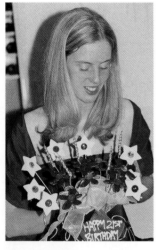

Me very reluctantly giving a speech at my birthday party.

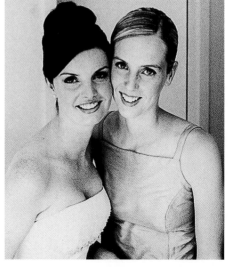

Sam, on her wedding day, and me as her bridesmaid.
(Photo courtesy Gregory's Photography)

I'm worried about my clothes being dirty after walking downtown today. I wanted to wash them straight away but my worker wouldn't let me, which made me really angry. I feel like I'm stupid and I'll never get anywhere in life.

Everyday people tell me that my perception about life and myself is wrong but I don't believe them. Margaret, another manager at the clinic, told me this morning they only make me eat things like flavoured yoghurt and don't allow me to measure things to show me that nothing will happen. But I don't see that. I think my body does change because of what I eat. I feel really bad for being such a mean person.

Sunday, 8 February 1998

I looked on the side of the yoghurt container this morning and it said it contained honey! That means more calories and proves that people have been lying to me by telling me that the only difference between plain and flavoured is the fruit.

I went out too much today. I was too busy and now I'm getting into lots of trouble in my head. I talk too much.

I like to write letters even though I shouldn't tell anyone how I feel or what I think. They can't say anything to change my mind anyway. I think people don't like me. No one has any reason to like me.

Monday, 16 February 1998

My toothbrush fell in the sink tonight so I washed it with soap, vinegar and boiling water. My workers told me that I couldn't get it any cleaner but I know it's no

*longer clean for me to use. Despite what I know, my
workers say I have to continue to use my dirty toothbrush.*

*My breakfast today had nuts in it. Nuts will add
more to the already overloaded with calories muesli –
so I took them out.*

*My hands are bleeding and really sore because
I washed my dishes, and other people's too, in really
soapy water. I probably made all my clothes dirty from
washing the dishes when the water splashed on me.
I wanted to put my clothes in the wash but I thought
I might get in trouble from my workers.*

Friday, 20 February 1998

*My ring fell off my finger during EP [Educational
Program] and landed on the floor and now I don't
want to put it back on because it's dirty. I kept thinking all day that I had to wash my hands because I'd
been touching dirty things. My wallet, the remote
control for the television, my bankcard, things that
had been on the floor, the oven, and a handle on a
door – the list goes on.*

*I threw out a bean and a carrot because they fell
out of my bowl and onto the table. My vitamins
fell onto the counter last night and I wouldn't have
them either.*

*I had a really tough time getting into my pyjamas
tonight because I feel my body is so big. I feel disgusting.*

Wednesday, 25 February 1998

*I went for a walk today and my camera case, lens cover
and film containers all fell on the footpath which*

made them dirty. My hands and face touched the camera, which is awful. I didn't want to touch any door handles while I was downtown especially with all the cuts on my hands from washing. Every time my cuts touched something while I was out I would start to worry about that bad disease.

I'm feeling rather discouraged right now about myself and about how other people see me. I always think I know exactly what other people think of me, because that's the way I see me. It's not a very nice view.

I now started to go out more often. Sometimes it was to have a meal and other times it was just to escape the house and the monotony of everyday life. Most of the time I would catch a ride with Bill, the Montreux driver. He was a gorgeous older man who loved his job. He drove us around in the silver Nissan van, back and forth all day and night, like a taxi driver. The drivers would rotate on an 8-hour shift but Bill was my favourite. I would go to Chapters, a big bookstore downtown, to sit in the comfy chairs in front of a beautiful, big open fireplace to read all night. Other times I would go to the Odeon with the old red vinyl seats and check out a movie. Usually Kornelia would come along. Shopping was another of our favourite activities, even though it was always just a window shop.

There was always something interesting happening in downtown Victoria depending on the season. The inner harbour is where all the action happened. The most incredible yachts would dock there during summer while jesters, fire-eaters, comedians, painters and buskers would sporadically set up shop for the next few months to entertain the holiday crowd. Victoria, although a small town, was always bursting at the seams during summer.

History was around every corner and the town had a very English feel thanks to its double decker buses, horse drawn carriages, pubs, neat gradens and afternoon teas. I had time to discover that Victoria was originally home to native Indians called the Camosack. While Captain James Cook sailed close to modern day Victoria in 1788, it was the famous Hudson Bay Company that set up Victoria as a trading post and fort some fifty or so years later. As everyone in Victoria will tell you, it wasn't until 1858 that this little town really took off when gold was discovered on the mainland of British Columbia. With adventurers flocking from all over the world, Victoria was the only ocean port for the gold fields. While the grand old stone buildings remain, the hustle and bustle of the gold rush was long gone, apart from the crowds in summer.

Thursday, 26 February 1998

I feel really upset today. I feel like the more time I spend here the less chance I have of getting well. It's as if the thoughts will never change and my fears will never go away. I'm sure it's all my fault because I've done something wrong.

My stomach is bothering me so much right now. I'm feeling a lot of discomfort tonight after my last snack.

Wednesday, 4 March 1998

This morning I had to touch a door handle to get into the restaurant for breakfast. I then had to eat my

*toast with my fingers after touching the door handle.
That is so disgusting. I'm sure something will happen
to me because I touched the handle.*

*When I walk down the street I always see red
things and other dirty things and I think I will get dirty
or a disease from walking past them.*

*I think everyone is angry with me because they
think I'm useless and a very annoying person.*

Friday, 20 March 1998

*Tonight I have to eat a pretzel with cream cheese and
jam. I always feel like such a pig when I eat things like
that. I wonder, too, if going out to eat is going to ever
change my fears about eating. I'm not allowed to wash
my hands but I still believe and think about my germ
phobia. It seems like the more I try to tackle one fear
something comes up in my mind about another fear.
Imagine the high jump bar in the Olympics and when I
jump over one fear my anorexia keeps raising the bar.*

*I don't believe I can get over this anorexia. I can't
imagine not having these terrifying thoughts and not
having to live by such a rigid and structured routine in
order to think I'm safe.*

*I can't let anyone else know my fears because they
probably think I shouldn't have them anymore and
that I should be at a different stage in my recovery.
When they see I'm behind in my recovery, they probably dislike me even more.*

Sunday, 22 March 1998

*My workers were switched this morning, which was
hard. They replaced Kristine with Janice because Janice*

was too tired to work at the Mansion. I'm obviously less important. I'm so sure everyone around here doesn't like me. I think everyone is disappointed in me.

Kristine had a personality that lit up any room or situation. A free spirit living life to the beat of her own drum, she was an incredible example of a happy soul. I spent many of my darkest moments with this incredibly strong Canadian woman. She cried with me, shared a very rare smile with me and genuinely cared for me. This curly blonde in her mid-30s was full of bright ideas and distractions. Kristine coined a whole new book of words which became a secret language between us and to this day there are phrases that are a part of my vocabulary that bring a smile to my face. I'm often asked why I'm smiling and all I can say is 'Kristine'.

Tuesday, 24 March 1998

I had trouble not being allowed to wash my hands. I always wanted to wash my hands today but my workers wouldn't let me. It's really hard not being able to wash my hands!

When I came home from the movies tonight, my head told me to throw my clothes in the dirty washing basket. My worker stopped me saying I had to hang them up and wear them tomorrow to prove I won't catch a disease from 'dirty' clothes. The rule at Montreux is I must wear my clothes more than once before washing them. That's really hard for me. My head is driving me crazy saying something terrible will happen if I don't wear freshly washed clothes every time.

Thursday, 26 March 1998

I went to get weighed this morning and I think Margaret told me that my weight hadn't changed just to keep me happy. But I feel so big and so enormous. I don't understand how I could not have gained weight when I look so ugly and fat.

Sunday, 29 March 1998

I think people here must hate me because I hate who I am. I think my room-mates are angry with me because they probably think I'm annoying. I feel bad for enjoying people's company and for laughing with my carer, Talya. People probably think I'm fine because I don't explain what's going on in my head. I'm afraid to tell people how I feel because they'll be disappointed in me or think less of me.

Tuesday, 31 March 1998

Peggy called to tell me that I'm not allowed to obsessively wash my hands any more. She said I can't act on the thoughts in my head. I don't know how to go against the things my head tells me because I'm so afraid of what it says.

I try because people tell me I have to try. However, if I were by myself I know I couldn't go against my head. It's too strong at the moment.

The fact I have all these beliefs and thoughts makes me feel hopeless. I feel like I've failed and I'll disappoint people if I tell them how I really, really feel. I'll tell you, my diary, how I feel. I feel like a BIG waste of time.

Wednesday, 1 April 1998

The spoon that I usually use to measure the food with was missing so I had to use a different one that was clearly bigger. This really bothered me.

I had trouble not being allowed to wash my hands. Sometimes there are things I want to touch but I can't because I know I'm not allowed to wash my hands. I've decided not to touch anything I think is dirty which rules out touching most things!

It was hard when I went downtown today because I kept seeing blood on things that I was touching. It really scares me. My head is still telling me those threats too about that blood disease that kills people!

I worry about my family so much. I wish I were there to protect them. What if my family doesn't like me? What if they think I'm mean and I'm just a disappointment to them?

Thursday, 2 April 1998

I feel out of control today. I don't see what other people tell me they see. It's a horrible feeling.

Anorexia is still putting all those threats in my mind. I find it hard to keep fighting it. I feel like crying. I feel I've upset other people and now they all hate me. I went into a session today thinking I can't tell my counsellor Colin anything because he's tired of hearing the same old stuff come out of my mouth.

I'm afraid I will never be free of this anorexia – that no matter how hard people try; it's somehow all my fault. Other people will get well. They deserve to get better but I don't.

Saturday, 4 April 1998

My worker didn't say anything about my food meas-
urements this morning so I actually put less in my
bowl. But no matter how much I put in the bowl it
seems too much. I could put nothing in there and
it would be too much.

I feel so alone. My worker this morning didn't really
seem to know what to do or say so I felt as though
I had to do everything by myself. It's hard to do things
for myself and to do what I'm supposed to do but I'm
so scared of not having someone helping me. It's hard
to be strong and go against my head on my own.

Sunday, 5 April 1998

It was hard to make today's snack after having less
yesterday. I felt like crying all afternoon and tonight.

I didn't want to go to the video store today because
all those videos have been touched by other people
and are so dirty. They must be covered in germs.

My head has been saying all those threats about
my family dying again! I'm trying to fight the threats
but it's hard. I feel very alone. I can't say anything to
anyone.

Wednesday, 8 April 1998

So many things scared me today. I left Richmond
House and I had to transport all my things up four
flights of stairs into my old apartment at St Charles.
I'm going onto partial care soon and Margaret and
Peggy want me to be up here where there are more
people for support. I put all my clothes into garbage
bags and other bags that I didn't think were clean.

I thought my hands were so dirty and I felt I had to keep washing them. Then my hands started to bleed and this really scared me.

I feel really lost.

I wanted to try partial care because I needed to test myself to discover my capabilities. This could only happen, I was told, if I moved back to St Charles so I could have more people around me for support. I jumped at the chance to move. The people I loved no longer lived there. A new generation of Richmond Housers had moved in and all the inspiration the house had once given me was now gone. My work there was done.

Part of the expectations of going onto partial care, and eventually 'off-care', was becoming more self-sufficient. This meant I couldn't use the 'driver' to catch a ride here and there, so I took to the streets on foot. Everything was quite close to where I lived in Victoria. Downtown was only a 20-minute walk and it was a walk I will remember for the rest of my life. I often varied my route and would stop by the beach on the way. Sometimes I would take Rockland Avenue, a windy road lined with huge oak trees and regal old timber and brick mansions. I loved walking this road in the fall. The leaves would turn the most amazing shade of red and burnt orange in autumn and I would walk on the footpath and scrunch them beneath my feet. This road would take me through a little village on Cooke Street, full of cafés and homeware stores. It was simply divine, like something out of an old *Murder She Wrote* mystery.

My other route was down St Charles Street (otherwise

referred to by all the Montreux residents as Cardiac Hill). This road wasn't windy but steep and straight. It took you to the beach and a magnificent view of the mountains across the water. On my journey this way I would pass baseball fields with kids throwing balls, Thrifty's supermarket with the slogan 'the smiles in the bag for you' and stunning beachside houses. Either route was breathtakingly beautiful.

Partial care was an enormous challenge and turned out to be so much harder than I expected it to be. I had gone from 24-hour care to 8-hour care. I was on my own during the day and had a care worker with me at night, but nothing had really changed from the day I had someone beside me all the time. I didn't miraculously feel better and decide I was fine on my own. Things got a whole lot worse. I felt like I was drowning.

Friday, 10 April 1998

I got really bad news today. Peggy rang me and said that my Poppa is really sick. He's got lung cancer and has only a few days to live. How will I cope with this? I feel like vomiting. I'm so upset about Poppa. I want to be able to help him. I feel powerless and helpless. It hurts so much.

I called Poppa and spoke to him for 3 hours. It turns out he's been sick for almost 2 years. I wasn't told because everyone thought I would leave and go back home to be by his side. I would have to!

Monday, 13 April 1998

I had an awful day. I feel really lost and so alone. I don't want to be by myself any more. I don't think I can deal with my anorexia any more. I don't think I can stop the terrible thoughts in my head and I don't think I can fight them all by myself.

My hands are really sore again from all my obsessive hand washing. I know my hands will get worse because I've been washing them more and more. I know I shouldn't wash them so much but I have to because they're so dirty.

I'm afraid of going to the bathroom and showering by myself because of my rituals and fears. What if I disobey my thoughts and something happens to someone in my family? I will be responsible for some terrible disaster.

I feel pretty huge right now. I just got changed for bed and I can see how big I've become, I don't like it. I'm so afraid and I feel as though I want to run away and hide from everyone around me and everything I have to deal with. I don't feel strong right now.

Tuesday, 14 April 1998

Poppa died today.

I didn't want to make my snacks today. It was such a battle because I feel so guilty, bad and ugly because I'm choosing to put on weight by measuring my food out properly. I want to put less in my mug and bowl. I don't need this food.

People have told me they would be here for me. So far, I don't think anyone has lived up to that promise. I want to run away. I feel lost as though everyone has deserted me.

Everyone expects me to be fine and to not think

all these terrible things about myself, my weight, my rituals, everything! I had a big struggle today with not being allowed to wash my hands. I didn't feel strong enough to fight the voices in my head so I gave in and now my hands are really sore.

Eating out tonight with my worker didn't help at all. The chicken was covered in sauce that probably had hundreds of calories in it. I felt I shouldn't be allowing myself to eat such a thing. It scared me and I sat and worried about it a lot when I came home. It worried me when the waitress came to serve our table because she had open cuts on her hands. I think she infected the chopsticks when she touched them and so I had no choice but to use the fork which I'm sure was dirty. What disease have I caught now?

I worry about my family because I think something terrible will happen to them, I have these dreams that one person in my family will die of AIDS or be hit by a car. Mum was murdered in one dream. They're so real.

My Poppa Clarke died the same day I went on partial care in 1998. I wanted to go home to Melbourne to see him but the clinic didn't want me to go as they thought it would set back my recovery. It was so hard as the family were all together supporting each other and I was on my own. They had known he was sick for a long time but I was only told a few days before he died so I would have a chance to talk to him. He told me wonderful stories of when he was young about the funny things he did with his brothers. It was a surreal experience because the whole time I was thinking this is the last time I'll ever speak with him. At the end of the conversation I said goodbye and he replied, 'It's not goodbye. I'll see you later.' He died four days later. He was seventy-six.

I cried for days. I felt sick and I couldn't eat or sleep. I was so angry. Angry that I hadn't been told he was sick, angry he was dying and angry because I hadn't only been robbed of the past five years of my life, education, boys and social life but I had also lost what would have been the last five years of my life and relationship with my grandfather. I had grown up with him and I adored him. It's now hard to remember the last moment I saw him or the last thing I said to him in person.

Wednesday, 15 April 1998

It's the anniversary of the Titanic disaster. It's funny how I remember a date like that. Maybe it's because I'm also a disaster.

I hated my old apartment at the top of St Charles, it brought back too many bad memories of my first days at Montreux. So I moved down to the basement today to share a room with Sarah and her crazy cat, Marley. I don't like living down here in the basement. It's so dark, small, messy and horrible. I really, really don't like it here. I can't live here for long. I want to run away. I feel like everything is just coming at me all at once.

Everyone is mad and disappointed with me. It's so hard not to wash my hands so I give in to the voices and scrub away. My hands are so sore now. I'm also finding it really hard to prepare my meals properly.

Thursday, 16 April 1998

Mum and Dad arrived today. We're going to light a candle in a church for Poppa. It's so nice to have them here with me at such a hard time. I feel guilty because Mum has had to leave Nanny to visit me.

Saturday, 18 April 1998

My groceries were delivered today and the nutritional information was blacked out so I couldn't see how much fat, sugar and calories they contained. I always want to choose the food I think has the least amount of calories. I don't need to put on more weight.

Sunday, 19 April 1998

Today was really hard because Peggy took my evening worker away to make me do everything on my own. I think everyone must hate me! Everyone expects me to be fine.

Thursday, 23 April 1998

My parents have just left after visiting me for a week. I feel guilty because I'm mean to my parents. I love them so much and I can't deal with thinking I've been selfish or ungrateful! I worry about them travelling home to Australia because the plane might crash and it will be my fault.

I had a difficult time today measuring my snacks and washing my hands. All the reasons why I want to wash my hands make sense to me – such as protecting my parents from a disaster – so I find it really hard to go against my head.

I find it exhausting trying to fight my thoughts all day by myself. I feel that everyone around me has all these expectations of me. Everyone expects me to be perfect and to not have problems. I feel as if I'm expected not to be afraid of anything because I'm on partial care. It scares me a lot being by myself.

I'm scared of myself. I don't want to be alone with my head and its orders of all the things I must do to stop awful things happening to my family. I find it hard to go against my head all by myself so I guess things will never change. What if I can't do this by myself and I will never get better? I don't feel like I can fight my head right now. Sometimes I feel so desperate I just want to run away. I want to run and run but I don't know where I would run! I feel so alone.

Partial care continued to be a real test for me. At times I felt I had got a little bit better but this radical change brought up all my fears. I became so focused on measuring my meals as I felt my body continue to balloon. My time on partial care was a succession of meals, frustration, fear and the never-ending handwashing.

Friday, 24 April 1998

I don't think anyone here likes me because they find me annoying. I don't believe them when they say they love me. Why should they? They're just lying to make me feel better.

I put too much cereal in my bowl this morning. When I'm measuring the right amount of food into my bowl I actually feel as if I'm putting in more. It makes me feel like I'm greedy and I'm choosing to gain weight!

I asked Mary, one of the other patients, to help me measure my yoghurt and she made me put so much more in than I wanted. It made me so mad. Now I feel really bad asking her for help. If I hadn't asked some-one to help I could have eaten less yoghurt.

I don't feel like I can cope beating anorexia all by myself. I feel overwhelmed.

Monday, 27 April 1998

I feel guilty asking for help. If I ask for help with my meals then I'm asking for more to eat and therefore asking to put on weight. I'm sure my weight keeps going up and up because I see my rolls of fat and I feel bigger!

I saw dirty things on the ground when I went for a walk down town. I'm so terrified of catching some disease from all the germs. I have to dodge around things, which makes my walk so much longer.

It feels like my head takes over and I can't stop it and I get into trouble if I go against it.

Wednesday, 29 April 1998

I feel bad for going out to lunch today. I ate pasta and tofu, which I'm sure was cooked in oil. Now I'm really afraid that I'm going to put on so much weight from eating such a huge meal. I think Justin, one of the counsellors, expects me not to be scared of eating out. Truth is, I'm terrified.

When I went for a walk today I saw my reflection in a window. I looked so big I could have been pregnant, that's how big I am. My hands are really sore and I can't stop washing them. I wash them more than I did when I was on full care. I have so many reasons to wash my hands.

Saturday, 30 May 1998

I feel so guilty for not going out for a walk today or doing very much. Maybe I wouldn't look so huge if I walked more and lost some weight. I feel the food just stays inside me when I eat – it never escapes.

I picked up the phone tonight to call for help from a worker but I just couldn't dial the number. I didn't think I was allowed to ring someone. I think I have to fix all my problems, and get through everything, by myself.

I'm still having a lot of trouble washing my hands. I can't seem to see through what I think. I feel like my hands are always dirty – that I'm always dirty – and that I have to wash all the time.

I'm a fighter and I will fight but I don't know if I can make it.

Friday, 5 June 1998

Today was extremely difficult. I went out for a sundae with Kirsten and Will. I've had my head shouting at me about the amount of calories I consumed. Now I can't eat for the rest of the day. The sundae was huge and I can't believe I ate it. I feel so guilty about it and I'm convinced that I'm already stacking on the kilos because of that sundae.

Will spent his summers playing professional golf and the rest of the year working with eating disorder sufferers.

I wasn't sure about Will when I met him in my first
month at Montreux. In his mid-twenties, Will was one of
the funnier carers and spent most of the time kidding
around. So when he turned up in my room at the Mansion and announced that he was my worker for that day,
I wasn't really sure what to think. My 'head' took an
instant dislike to him for various reasons. He was on my
'to cull' list for quite some time.

A little later in my program, Will arrived on my
doorstep while I was at Richmond House and again
declared himself as my worker. I had no choice about the
matter and decided to make the most of it. From then on,
Will became one of my favourite people to work with.
He taught my friend Becca and I how to play golf. We
would set off to the driving range in his old metallic blue
car with fuzzy dice hanging from the rear-vision mirror
that we named Lady Luck.

Will spent a lot of time with Becca and me in our
partial care days when we were in our low spiral and he
brightened our days.

Monday, 8 June 1998

*I'm so afraid of being left alone to deal with my
anorexia. I'm afraid everything will get out of control.
I keep all my fears, thoughts and feelings a secret
because telling people would be like letting them
down. Letting people know I need help is something
I just can't do! If I call Peggy she will be mad with me
and think I'm wasting her time. I feel guilty for still
being here in Canada. I feel pathetic and I'm sure
that's what other people think of me too. I see the
new patients and think how selfish I am to ask for help*

when Peggy and other counsellors must be so busy helping them.

It was hard when I put a dress on today. It felt tight and I looked so big in it, and it was a size large! I'm so scared I'm putting on weight. I'm so afraid that I'm becoming this huge obese person. It's so hard to do the things that people tell me to do in order to get better. As a result of getting better with food I feel like I'm putting on lots of weight.

I saw an old photograph of me the other day with the nasogastric tube and I know how much I never want to be like that again. I do want to be well so much but sometimes it seems just so impossible. It's such a hard fight and sometimes, no matter how hard I try, I just can't seem to change my thoughts. I get so afraid when people tell me to go against my thoughts because I fear the threats made by my head to my family and me.

I feel like a loser. I feel like I have a tug-a-war going on in my head. There's a part saying, 'Don't eat this, lose weight. Ignore every one, you'll always be like this.' Then there's a part that wants to ask for help, who wants to be well more than anything else in the world and who wants to do everything right and listen and talk to people.

Wednesday, 10 June 1998

Everyone hates me, I know it. I don't like myself so why would any one else like me? Peggy told me that next week I'll be off-care and I'll have to eat alone and now I'm scared that I'll want to skip my meals. I don't think of myself as a liar but I'm so afraid to tell anyone what

I'm thinking or feeling. I keep thinking that maybe if I just pretend everything is all right then they'll let me go home.

Peggy asked me today if I'm still behaving obsessively. She said it in such a tone that I didn't think I could answer her truthfully but I don't want to lie. She asked me why I'm acting like a wimp. I don't like to think of myself as a wimp, I'm just finding things really difficult right now. She also asked me why I had been phoning people. Firstly, she tells me to call her and other people whenever I need to then it seems to me like she was saying I shouldn't need to call people. I'm getting some very confusing messages here.

I see everyone else here and they all look so skinny and tiny and I feel like such a huge, FAT pig. I'm continuously eating and half the time it's food I don't even like. I'm afraid to eat what I enjoy to eat because it must have more calories in it, as if I'm not already big enough. I've been having trouble with my hand washing and with things around me being dirty.

Peggy called to say I had let [her daughter] Nicole down. I feel bad about this and I want her to know that I always try to give something back to those who give so much to me. I feel I'm a terrible person. I think Peggy and Nicole both hate me. I think I'm disappointing because I find it hard to follow my meal plan.

Nicole was Peggy's other daughter. She was the youngest and was simply stunning to look at. She was elegant and graceful and always smelt of sweet perfume. She was quite tall with long, wavy, light brown hair and blue eyes.

She had some of Peggy's physical features like her mouth and the shape of her face. I imagine Peggy would have looked just the same at Nicole's age. Nicole had suffered anorexia in her teens, recovered and had worked at Montreux since it opened. She was now twenty-eight and a 'sort of' counsellor. She took patients out and spent time with them at Montreux. She was almost ghostlike. She would come and go so often that a sighting of Nicole was quite treasured. She was also a photographer and would take the most amazing photos of the patients to send home as gifts for their parents. She was up-beat and creative.

I looked up to Nicole and over the period of my time at the clinic I formed quite a strong friendship with her. She invited me into her home and I spent Christmas with her and her little boy, Darius. We would take drives to find gorgeous locations for photoshoots and I would assist her on the shoots. I made piñatas for Darius' birthday party and watched him grow up.

Thursday, 11 June 1998

I get angry with myself for feeling the way I do. I find it hard to get past what my head says to me. I truly want to be free of my fears. I want to be normal. I want to be able to do what I want and to eat what I want, when I want.

Peggy told me I've lost weight and that I have to regain the weight plus some! So, on top of eating, I have to have the Ensure shakes which will make me gain even more weight. Even though Peggy says I need to put on weight, I don't want to put on weight!

Kornelia has now left Victoria to share a house with Charlie in England. I miss her so much.

**

I went off-care mainly because there weren't enough workers to cope with the number of clients at the clinic. Off-care meant I didn't have a care worker with me at all during the day, evening or night. I still had my counselling sessions during the week and I could call anyone from Montreux for support, but now the responsibility for fighting anorexia and following the program fell to me.

The transition from partial care to off-care was difficult and my health went downhill. I went through a really rough time when I stopped eating again and I lost a significant amount of weight. It got harder until I made a choice. I had come to a fork in the road of my recovery. Two paths lay ahead. One was to continue in my 'safe' alliance with my anorexia, the other was to put my trust in others even though I didn't believe in them most of the time. This became the defining moment of my illness. I got to the point where I had to see if there was something better out there and I just had to go through it the hard way.

I became almost bull-like and every little thing my negative mind frightened me with I would challenge with ten times the force than I ever had to fight it before. It was almost as if I was training for the Olympics of life. My training was constant; I fought every morning until late at night. That's not to say I didn't have hiccups along the way. I had days when I was just too tired from all the training and wanted to give up. It was these moments that gave me the strength to go on. I would think about where I had come from and think back to something that only a month ago had been so hard and was now much easier. I just had to believe in myself.

So much of the bloody hard work was done on my own. I had been through three different counsellors by this stage and had come to the point where I really needed someone to help me with the ME stuff and someone who had the time to stand beside me as I challenged the most frightening aspects of life – socialising, food, learning about myself and stepping back into life.

At this stage, being surrounded by other 'sick' people was not healthy for me. I was trying to understand life and hang onto it and Montreux was not a normal environment. It was like we were taken out of the world and wrapped up in cottonwool. I knew I wouldn't get the experiences and learn the things I needed to learn in that environment so I enrolled in a short photography course at Camosun College, an old and beautiful building sitting on top of a hill. I also began volunteer work with grades one and two at a local primary school. These things took my mind off the hard work that faced me when I got home.

Juliette, an off-care support counsellor, would catch the bus with me to the primary school, which was frightening at first but got much easier the more I did it until I got to the point when I could do it on my own. She would also pick me up when I had finished and we would spend an hour challenging my fears and talking about how I felt. Sometimes Juliette and I would go out to eat ice-creams and burgers – real meals from all different sorts of places. Basically, she would challenge me. If I didn't want to eat something at the apartment she would take me out to a restaurant or café to have it. Inevitably I would get back to my apartment and freak out and I would want to compensate by missing my next meal. By now, however, I was much better at asking for help and I would call

Juliette to work through how I was feeling. How was I to learn that everything in moderation was safe unless I tested myself to see if it was actually true? Again, like a bull, I put my head down and ran head first into what felt like a brick wall.

Juliette took me swimming, which was the first time I had been in a pool, public or private, in about eight years. I not only freaked out about wearing bathers in public but also being in what I considered to be germ-infested water. Again, the more we went swimming the easier it became for me. We would also go out for coffee or herbal teas in Victoria. Socialising seemed normal and I was afraid of what was considered to be normal by society. I was also afraid the staff at Montreux would consider me to be 'well' if they knew I could eat and socialise. Being 'well' on the outside meant they would no longer want to help me, or so my mind told me. I knew that inside I felt I wasn't close to being OK.

The staff at Montreux never seemed to really understand that I wasn't OK inside and when I would try to talk to someone about it all I would hear was, 'You should be past this by now.' Those comments always shook my brittle confidence and in response I vowed to keep my feelings to myself and pretend everything was fine just to make others happy. Juliette was the one person who knew how I felt and did everything she could to help me. I also had a few of my old workers help me get through this time. Linda would call me, visit me, and have me over at her house all the time. These were the people who kept me sane throughout this time.

Linda was simply amazing. I liked her the minute I met her as one of my care workers. She was so kind and intuitively understood the illness and all the pain that came with it. I always felt completely safe in her care. She was tall, blonde and in her late thirties when we met. As I progressed through the program, her home became a second home to me. It was full of antiques, was painted in warm yellows and sage greens and smelled of puppies because she always seemed to have a litter of lost or abandoned dogs living in her spare bedroom. There were cats, too, with all creatures living in perfect harmony together, sometimes up to twenty at once. Linda constantly challenged my condition and stood by me through everything. She gave me an escape from Montreux and invited me into her world.

One day, Peggy and Nicole decided they would now be my counsellors as Juliette was needed elsewhere. This was well meaning but wasn't really a good thing for me as they were rarely at the clinic and hardly ever in the country, which made them hard to contact. I felt even more isolated. Thankfully Juliette missed me and still managed to spend time with me on the side. Perhaps this is why I came to the conclusion that I needed to discover life outside Montreux and why I worked so hard to get to a point where I felt strong enough to try out Australia. I had been doing so much of this bloody hard work by myself. I had a spirit inside me that wouldn't be broken. I didn't feel like I fitted the Montreux mould any more. It was time to see what I could do.

Saturday, 11 July 1998

I've been skipping parts of my meals. I'm not having my fruit all the time and I don't always have my juice. I don't know what my yoghurt measurement is so

I just put in what I feel is right, which isn't always enough. I also don't have all my protein. If I'm having tuna I will just have one can instead of the one-and-a-half cans that I'm meant to, according to my meal plan. If I'm having chicken, I will pull off the bits I think are bad and leave a quarter of the food. I find that I have cut back on my food each time I prepare a meal.

I freak out that I'm going to put on weight when I'm already so fat. My roommate Becca is so thin. She can eat anything and she doesn't gain an ounce.

It's been about a month or so since I've been off-care and I know I'm not well right now. I don't feel strong enough to take over and control the thoughts in my mind.

I expect so much of myself and therefore I think others also have the same expectations of me. Kirsten said I should go for more walks and this made me feel like a BIG FAT PIG. So I want to walk all the time now. When Peggy asked me who wanted to go for a walk, my head or me, I said me. I wasn't telling the truth.

I made some great friends at Montreux, one in particular was Rebecca, or Becca as I called her. She was my roommate in Canada over the summer of 1998 and made the most impact on me. I moved in with her at the beginning of June and stayed there until November. We went through some really tough months together as we had both just moved from partial care to off-care. We used each other as support. Becca was from Florida in America and spoke with a southern drawl. Over time I picked up on her accent and soon spoke in a similar way.

Becca was nineteen when we met and she had so much going for her. She had a wicked sense of humour and was the brainiest kid on the block. She was gorgeous with her light brown hair, big blue eyes and crystal clear complexion. She became like a sister to me. We were inseparable. We passed the time doing puzzles, hanging in coffee shops, reading books, watching movies and sitting at Victoria's pretty inner harbour having philosophical conversations about the meaning of life. We shared our dreams with one another. I knew what she wanted to call her kids one day, if she ever got to have them, and she knew what I wanted to call mine. She was a gentle soul. An angel.

She came from a very loving and supportive family but in the end it wasn't enough for her. She had a heart of gold and no matter how she was feeling inside she would always smile and do something thoughtful to bring sunshine into the days of others. As I began to recover, Becca seemed to go backwards. She would say that anorexia was too powerful and controlling for her to battle against. It strained our friendship as I was trying so hard to move forward. Being around her was a constant reminder of what I was trying to leave behind. Becca began giving in to the thoughts that I was trying to fight and seeing someone do that made me question if I was right to keep pushing on.

Sunday, 26 July 1998

I feel extremely guilty for eating food like avocado and olive oil. I know I have to eat but I find it so hard.

Right now, for example, I feel huge and terrible for all the things I ate today. I feel like I'm eating so much food. I haven't been sleeping well at all. I'm tired and

I have a constant headache. I feel like I always have to go out for walks to compensate for all of the extra food I'm eating. Not only do I have to eat my entire regular meal plan but also I have to eat more because I'm still losing weight. I have a hard time comparing myself with other patients. They all look so skinny to me and I feel like a huge person. I feel lazy if I sit for too long. I don't feel like I can just sit down and relax because then I'll feel even bigger and gain even more weight.

Peggy, Kirsten, Colin and Nicole have all told me I can call whenever I need to talk to someone for help but I still don't think I can. I think I'm such a pain . . . a bother.

I feel like I've failed because I've had people helping me out with my meals. I know if I was by myself that I would not eat what I'm supposed to. Everyone suspects that I'm not eating all my food. I need someone to watch me so I can eat.

It's now 2 a.m. and I can't sleep. I want to call someone to talk about why I can't sleep but I don't think that I have the right to call anyone.

Friday, 31 July 1998

I can't take Peggy telling me to be a soldier and to stand up to my thoughts. Becca keeps telling me to smile. She makes me feel even worse about myself.

Peggy put me, then Becca, on the scales. She didn't let me see my weight but I'm sure I weigh much more than Becca. I weigh more than everyone else. It's always been that way. Peggy said I have to eat bananas and to have three huge tablespoons of mayonnaise with my tuna. Since I'm expected to do everything alone, I have decided not to do anything I'm told to do. I'm already big enough and I don't need more fat to make me bigger.

I'm so afraid of the things I think I'm expected to be over and when I get upset I'm told to stop crying like I'm not supposed to feel anything.

I'm scared to be alone right now but I don't want anyone with me either. I feel like a big failure. I don't think anyone would notice, let alone care, that I'm not eating everything I should be. I can't tell anyone about the other problems I have with obsessive behaviour because my counsellors have told me not to be scared and to not think those things. That way, they say, everything will OK. It's just like pretending that a problem doesn't exist. It's still there whether you address it or not!

Monday, 10 August 1998

I went out for lunch today and I think I should have stayed in my apartment to avoid the food. I had to eat an entire pizza and oily, greasy bread. This was a scary meal. I had a hard time deciding what to eat, as I couldn't figure out which one had fewer calories. I'm not happy about it! I'm not going to have my Ensure shakes tonight because I don't need to gain weight.

I've been trying so hard to do everything I've been told to do but I know everything just puts on weight. Peggy said when I put on weight she would decrease the food on my meal plan. I called her to talk about it but she didn't call me back. I think she doesn't want to talk to me.

Friday, 14 August 1998

I can't sleep. I'm stressing out about my life and panicking that I can't sleep. I feel like I'm going to throw up. My stomach has been so sore today and has been so big. I think it's because of my big scary meal plan, full of fat and excessive calories.

Please let me go to sleep.

Saturday, 15 August 1998

I can't sleep again tonight so I thought I should write in my diary. Today was hard because I ate all my snacks for the first time in a long while.

Peggy promised me that she would change my meal plan once I gained some weight. I know that I have put on so much weight but Peggy won't change my meal plan and I've started panicking so I will change my meal plan myself because nobody else will. I know that I'll gain even more weight if I eat my entire meal plan.

I don't want to disappoint people here, or myself for that matter. Peggy said she was ashamed of me because I promised I would do everything I was meant to do and I didn't. I feel bad about thinking I might have upset and disappointed her.

I feel really bad for calling Nicole on her mobile phone today. How selfish of me interrupting a busy person like that. I put myself first way too much.

I've been told in the long run that it's better for me to do what I'm supposed to do and stick to the program even if I feel horrible and frustrated. Continuing to follow anorexia's ways will get me nowhere in a big hurry but it's easier said than done. The staff here make out that defeating anorexia is a breeze when it's really hard. I'm scared of trying to fight by myself.

Saturday, 22 August 1998

I don't understand how Peggy can say that I'm underweight. I don't see why I should have to gain weight. It makes no sense to me.

I feel like getting down on the floor and doing sit ups or going for a long walk or a jog. I need to burn off all the weight I'm putting on from the extra food I'm eating.

Today I had a huge tuna sandwich with way too much mayonnaise and butter on it. I also had an avocado and oil followed by two shakes later on in the day.

I don't think I can keep fighting this battle with anorexia. Peggy told me I shouldn't be acting this way, which makes me feel like a failure.

Saturday, 5 September 1998

Mum and Nanny arrive tomorrow to see me, which will be great. I think it's good for Nanny to get away after nursing Poppa for so long.

They plan to stay for a week before leaving for a month-long holiday in Europe. While they're with me we're going to do the tourist thing for a week and even go whale watching.

1999

Monday, 15 February 1999

Well, I have a new meal plan and it's so different to my old one. Kirsten gave me the choice; stay with my old meal plan and stay sick or try the new one. I've been stressing out for a week but I've decided I'm going to do it and I'm sure that it won't be as bad as my fears make it out to be. The meal plan has scary food on it such as pudding, cheesecake and ice-cream. I don't want fear to control me. I would rather control it, or better still, get rid of it. I want so much to live FREE. I want to be WELL.

I think I should be home by now. I see patients who arrived at Montreux after me going home for visits and, in some way, I feel like a failure.

What's the key? Is it my fault that I haven't figured it out? Of course, it's my fault! Some people tell me it's about letting go so why can't I let go?

I'm not thinking or saying that things haven't changed. I know that so much has changed but I now feel stagnant and I fear this is as far as I can go. Maybe being completely well is not an option for me, which is a thought that scares me. I want to eat what I want the way a child would. Can I ever feel like that, I wonder?

Friday, 19 February 1999

I had a difficult time with the puddings today because I saw the list of ingredients by accident. It bothered me what was in there but I continued eating them. I really wish that I didn't care what was in food. I want to be able to see that things don't make a difference, just like everyone tells me. I want to just get rid of all my fears and believe what people tell me but I continue to have these thoughts in my head. Why? It must be my fault I guess.

I wish I was more honest with Scott, my new counsellor, and Colin as well as the others when I say I don't like the taste of certain food. What I'm trying to say is that I'm scared of eating the food. I know I shouldn't expect people to do things for me but I do want them to push me to recovery because I can't do it by myself.

Sometimes when I'm out, as hard as it feels, I wish someone would tell me to eat something scary to challenge me. That way I know if I'm getting somewhere, even though it feels really hard. If I never push myself, I'll never change. And all this inner strength that Kirsten says I have, well, I wish I had more of it so I could be more courageous!

I think I shouldn't even write these thoughts in my diary. I don't want to be thought of as a negative person. I want to think that maybe people do like me and that maybe I'm not so bad instead of always thinking how annoying, boring and selfish I am.

Sunday, 28 February 1999

I feel really alone today. Actually, I feel alone a lot of the time. I find it really hard being off-care. I wish I had someone I knew I could talk to because I still have difficulties with many things. I feel like I always have to be the good girl, cause no trouble and put on a brave face.

I feel I've been here too long and I fear people resent me for that. I wish I was well. I wish anorexia never happened to me. I find it really hard to see myself completely well, completely happy. That's something I've never felt and is so foreign to me.

I find it really hard to change my thought patterns and beliefs. On top of that, I have these expectations of myself to be well NOW and that I should have changed my mind. It's my fault that I'm not well. I lack the knowledge and ability to ever be well.

Friday, 12 March 1999

I've just read over my diary entries from when I first arrived in Canada and, wow, how my whole world has changed for the better. I still have trouble with things but in different ways and to different degrees. Right now, I'm working on challenging myself with all sorts of things such as going out for ice-cream, KFC and eating red meat, all the food that really frightens me.

Today I did something that I'm so proud of – I ate a chocolate and I survived. You know what else? It tasted really good. Sure, I panicked afterwards but it hasn't occupied my mind all day. Actually I'm proud of myself for challenging myself like that. It may seem a small thing, but it's really a big deal to me.

Thursday, 18 March 1999

Everyday I wake up, I'm grateful to think that I prob- ably wouldn't be here breathing today if it weren't for

Montreux and my family. I know I was so blessed in coming to Montreux. People who love me unconditionally surround me. Sometimes I think everyone hates me but those thoughts are fewer these days. Becca is one of my best friends. She is so smart, kind and thoughtful. I'm glad I have such a good friend like her. And then of course there's Kornelia, who's moved from England and lives in France right now, but I keep in contact with her and we talk often. Then there's Nicole, such a good friend. I love her very much. She has given so much love and support. She's an inspiration to me and I admire her so much.

Kirsten and Peggy – their strength, knowledge and understanding amaze me. Noah, Margaret, and all my care workers, are such kind people who have never once given up on me. I could never have imagined being where I am today when I first arrived here nearly three years ago. I'm sure I will get well. I will be free. I don't have very much belief in myself but the people around me do!

I struggle with the length of time I've been here. I know that everyone takes his or her own time to recover. Peggy and Nicole told me that it doesn't matter how long it takes as long as I'm moving forward every day in my recovery. Nicole tells me, it's better to take it slowly and do it right, than go fast and relapse.

I try to keep myself busy so I don't have too much time to think. Some days I feel the negativity in my mind stronger than other days. It's been quite strong lately.

Sunday, 4 April 1999

Well here it is – Becca's birthday, Easter and a sad day too. I feel guilty for what I have put my family through. I feel bad that even now I don't feel strong enough to go home. I think I'm a bad daughter. I only wish I could see any goodness that I hold inside. I wish I was free of this anorexia that has been holding me captive so long.

Monday, 12 April 1999

I'm very homesick for my family at the moment. I miss them terribly. I haven't seen Jordan, James and Sam in more than two years. I long to hug them. I haven't seen Dad in a year and Mum since she came with Nanny last September. I long to hug Dad and Mum. I hope they always know and remember how much I love them.

My relationship with my Nanny remained as strong as ever during my time at Montreux. She would send me a letter every week updating me on life at home. Every word of every letter was full of love and happiness, even though my Poppa was sick for much of the time. I kept each letter and I have them very carefully stored away to this day. They are like a journal of life in Australia and of the family that I missed.

Very rarely would I reply to a letter from Nanny. I stayed in touch with my extended family at the beginning of my treatment but I slowly found I was so engrossed in my illness that it was too hard for me to communicate with anyone outside my immediate world. I felt guilty for not writing back to Nanny.

Tuesday, 4 May 1999

It's about 1.30 a.m. and I can't sleep so I've turned to my diary for help.

I think I'm a pretty selfish person. I don't give enough to others such as money, kindness and compliments. Is my heart bad, I ask myself? My family tell me I've been so kind all my life but I don't remember being kind as a child. I don't remember ever being nice. I just think how selfish I've been in doing everything for myself.

I want to be good. I want to be kind, loving, giving, all things that make a good heart and good spirit. There's so much for me to learn about life and so much for me to experience. I know I have so much work to do here on Earth. There's a reason behind things. I don't know the reason for this anorexia happening to me but maybe it was meant for me to learn.

Sometimes I get angry when I think of how much I have missed in my life such as my family and friends. I get so extremely frustrated with myself for being here three years later, still working on things and struggling through things.

Saturday, 8 May 1999

I panicked today thinking I'll never be good enough. I think I've done everything wrong my entire life. I want to be kind to everyone. I feel like I'm a terribly selfish person. I don't give enough to others, I don't do enough for others and I don't love enough. I'm constantly asking myself if I'm being kind enough.

I used to feel like I had no future but I now know I

have so much to live for. I look forward to being able to help others someday and to being married and having my own family. I love kids. I think they are so wonderful, innocent and carefree. I look forward to being carefree one day.

Sometimes I fear that my problems will never go away because I've been here too long. It troubles me knowing so many suffering people need to be here but can't get in because there aren't enough places for everyone.

There is so much that I have to learn but at least I've got time on my side.

Sunday, 9 May 1999

Today is Mother's Day and I've had my mind on Mum quite a bit. I miss her. I miss my family very much and I think of them always. I hope they always know in their hearts how much I love them. Holidays and celebrations are especially hard times to be away as they're so family oriented. I miss Australia but I only want to go back when I'm ready and strong enough. I want to travel to Italy someday, Tuscany. It sounds so beautiful there. This world sure is a beautiful place, if we look at the good things and keep things simple.

My Dad told me the world is amazing and wonderful when we keep it simple but we complicate it so much. Sometimes when I'm walking or looking out my window, I marvel at how beautiful this world is.

It wasn't until July of 1999 that television and I met again. My parents had been staying in Canada for a few months to spend time with me. We were planning to go to Seattle then Los Angeles for a week or so, which was a huge challenge for me. I was stepping away from the safety net of the clinic and I was scared.

At this point Ray Martin had left *A Current Affair* to work on his own documentaries and specials. Producer Margie Bashfield called to say Ray wanted to film my family and me in LA to start work on a one-hour special. Again, I didn't want Ray and his camera crew to come over because it seemed all too much for me at once. However, I was talked into it and my family and the TV crew all met in LA.

Despite my initial reservations, it turned out to be a really fun week in spite of the hard moments and challenges. We went to Disneyland, the Chinese Theatre in Hollywood, Universal Studios and relaxed at Santa Monica. We shopped a lot and ate out every night. It gave me a taste of life and reminded me of all the things my anorexia kept me from doing. My parents left for Melbourne in August. I was alone again.

In September I got a call from Ray Martin in Sydney asking if he could finish my story in Canada. I was stunned. I hadn't finished my program at Montreux, nor was I anywhere near finishing my journey of recovery. I felt they were asking me to do something that I just couldn't do. I also thought that since I'd only been with them a couple of months earlier, they could give me a little bit more time until they came again.

I kept saying no and they kept saying yes with different people calling (including my family) trying to convince me to say yes. I couldn't understand why they wouldn't try to understand how I felt and think about what I wanted. It was then that I started to feel like I was just a ratings winner and all that ever really mattered was that the

'Bronte Show' did better than before. It dawned on me that perhaps the reason they were pushing so hard to film me was the need to do a little better in the ratings. These thoughts plagued me and I spent many sleepless nights angry and hurt over the whole thing. I kept wishing I had never had anything to do with the media.

In the end I said yes to Ray and Channel Nine. They brought my sister Sam, who I hadn't seen in three years, and my Mum over to Canada in November 1999. That's why I said yes. Seeing them made the television experience a lot easier to handle.

Christmas of 1999 was a terrible time for me. I was really struggling with my anorexia and I was mentally exhausted after my parents' trip and all the filming with Channel Nine. I felt so alone and very distant in my little room in Canada. I didn't know where I belonged anymore. My family wanted me to come home but I wasn't sure if I was ready to face such a huge challenge. I was scared of going home. At the same time, an investigation into Montreux by the Canadian medical authorities had begun and the word was that the clinic was going to be shut down. It was an awful time and I didn't know how this would affect my future or if I even had one.

Opinion on the treatment at the Montreux Clinic was split. On one side you had former patients and supporters who claimed Peggy Claude-Pierre was a saviour devoted to helping sufferers and their families. She was running the last chance saloon, and patients loved her. On the other side of the fence were the medical establishment who claimed she was an amateur who didn't really know what she was doing and couldn't possibly have a success rate of almost 100 per cent. There were claims of stories of unhappy former patients, of a lack of proper medical care and force-feeding. Some critics even likened the clinic to a cult.

Part Four

Coming Home

2000

Monday, 21 February 2000

I've made a huge decision! I've decided to go home for a visit. I'm still in the middle of planning the trip but I hope to be able to go in March so I can be there for Mum and Jordan's birthday. I've also heard a whisper from Dad that Scott is going to propose to Sam in mid-March. I want to be there for that. I'm excited at the thought of going home but I'm also so scared.

Tuesday, 7 March 2000

I'm sitting on my bed looking out my window at the snow-capped Olympic Mountains. They're so beautiful when it's cold. I'm going home to Melbourne today. It's just a visit, but I'm going home. I can't believe it. I feel like I'm dreaming. I have butterflies in my stomach. I don't know if I can do this. Oh . . . gotta go. Bill has just called. He's here to drive me to the bus.

I often dreamed about returning home during my treatment in Canada. I was so terribly homesick when I first arrived that all I wanted to do was go home. As time passed so did the homesickness. I didn't miss Australia, I missed my family. Australia to me was a place of bad memories and I became terrified that if I ever returned, those bad memories would come flooding back and become an awful reality. I felt safe in Canada and there was a long period where I felt it was the only place I would be able to stay. So the thought of returning home seemed impossible. In fact, I became quite sure that I would never be well enough to go home so I gave up on the thought completely.

As time meandered by in Canada, the question of when I was coming home to visit was often raised during conversations with my family. I would always have a reason why I couldn't come and the reason never changed. I just wasn't ready. I think my family were often offended because they thought I didn't want to be with them. The truth is I missed my family terribly but I had my counsellors at the clinic telling me that if I wanted to get better then perhaps I shouldn't go to Australia.

As I got stronger and more independent I started discovering things for myself. In my fourth year at Montreux, one thing I realised was that I had a really strong desire to go home for a visit. I was so excited to make that decision for myself. I told one of my counsellors, 'This is something I'm terrified of but I need to do it to challenge myself.' Once I'd made the choice, I became excited about my decision. I knew I wasn't ready to go for a long period so I planned to go for a couple of weeks.

It was a frosty March morning and the fog made everything seem so romantic, like one of those moments when time stands blissfully still. I looked at the mountains and ocean through my window, a magnificent view that had never seemed so endless before this day in 2000. Life felt surreal. I was absolutely terrified, I was shaking, yet I was also excited. Was I really about to venture out into the 'real world' and leave everything I knew to be safe behind me?

I closed the door to my suite at seven in the morning, took a deep breath, and met a group of smiley faces at the bottom of the stairs. They told me they would miss me terribly and couldn't wait until I got back to hear the tales of my trip. Also waiting for me was a television crew hired by Channel Nine to record my departure. The only notable absentees were Peggy and her daughter Nicole. Bill, Becca and Linda drove me to the bus depot in the heart of downtown Victoria.

I had taken this bus trip before but it had never taken so long as it did that morning. The bus travelled up the island from Victoria to the port of Sidney where the ferries docked. From here the ferry took me across the icy-cold seas of the Strait of Georgia to the city of Vancouver on the Canadian mainland. While the ferry ride is one of the most spectacular voyages anyone could experience, I had become immune to the natural beauty because I had taken the crossing many times. But this day was different. My senses were heightened as if I were on some kind of drug. It felt like I was experiencing the ferry crossing – and the incredible natural beauty around me – for the first time. By the time I reached Vancouver airport I had been travelling for 6 hours and was beginning to feel tired. I think I was tired from all the thinking rather than the travelling.

I flew home via Hong Kong which must be one of the longest routes to Australia from Canada! As I settled into my seat, I remember thinking, 'It won't take that long.'

We had an Australian captain on our Cathay Pacific flight who proudly announced, 'Our flight to Hong Kong today will be 15 hours.' I looked out the window and thought, 'Let me off this thing!'

Soon after take-off, I got out my Discman CD player, reclined my seat and let the sounds of Canadian singer songwriter, Sarah McLachlan soothe me. Her music gave me a feeling of safety, her voice wrapping itself around me like a warm, comforting security blanket. I closed my eyes and for a brief moment it was as if I was back in my room in Victoria, and I wasn't really leaving Canada behind.

Reality hit me when the food service began, forcing me to switch off Sarah. I hadn't seen so much food in a long time. Dinner seemed to be about eight courses long and I started to feel frightened and overwhelmed. Despite my fear I not only didn't freak out at the food, I actually ate a chicken dish, some fruit and chocolate. What a contrast to the flight going the other way more than three years earlier! I could finally enjoy food.

There was a slight delay in transferring planes at Hong Kong – actually it was more of a major 4-hour delay due to a malfunction. This sort of hiccup, commonly known in my family as 'Jan's luck', had somehow rubbed off onto me. (Mum's luggage always seems to go missing when she flies.) The worst thing about the delay, apart from the complimentary weak cordial to tide us over at four in the morning, was that it gave me more time to mull over what I was flying towards.

The plane finally got it together and was scheduled to land in Melbourne at 1 p.m., eight hours away. I was dealing with the entire travelling across the world thing on my own particularly well and actually enjoying the adventure until a very friendly flight attendant approached me to tell me we were getting close to Melbourne. She said that as I had a camera crew waiting for me in the terminal I had to be the first off the plane. Great! She also said I needed to sit at the very front of the plane.

I was moved to the only empty seat at the front of business class, right next to Paul Keating. Our former prime minister didn't seem too pleased to see me invading his personal space. I felt like I was in the way and started feeling nervous. This was topped off by the first officer announcing, 'We are now approaching Melbourne.' I started to cry. I felt like I was in a dream sequence when I finally saw the houses in dot form below me and the city skyline on the horizon. I had to pinch myself to make sure it was real.

Paul Keating and I were to be first off the plane. While we were waiting for the door to open a man standing behind me asked, 'Are you a star? Are you a star? Do you make movies?' I told him no, but as soon as the door opened Paul Keating was taken to the VIP exit, leaving me staring at the waiting camera crew. The sight excited the man behind me who shouted. 'You are a star! Why didn't you tell me?' Truly bizarre.

Thursday, 9 March 2000

Here I am in Melbourne. The flight over was so long and tedious, but I still enjoyed it. It was so wonderful to see everyone again. I didn't want a fuss at the airport but there they were, Mum, Dad, the boys, Nanny and Aunty Gail with banners and balloons for me. I felt so loved. I'm so lucky to have my family. The dogs Muffin and Mac remembered me as soon as I walked in the door and I have already made friends with Bob,

*Muffin's little puppy. Today was fantastic but exhaust-
ing. I can't wait to see what tomorrow brings.*

I knew my family, some of whom I hadn't seen in three
years, would be waiting at Melbourne airport for me. As
it turned out, my Mum, Dad, Nanny, Jordan, James and
the camera crew, my now adopted family, were all there.
As I came through the exit doors at the international
terminal I saw them all there shouting, crying, waving
banners and holding balloons. My emotions, and my
stomach, were churning and for a moment I thought of
turning around and heading straight back on the plane.
I'd wanted a low-key, no-fuss arrival so the over-the-top
Cullis welcoming committee was a bit embarrassing and
overwhelming. But within an instant I was struck by a
wonderful feeling of happiness. This was my family; the
people I loved dearly and they were here for me. I had
seen Mum only four months before and Dad seven
months earlier, but hugging my brothers for the first time
in so many years was an experience that words can't
describe.

As we left the airport and headed to the car, the next
thing to hit me was the extreme heat. I hadn't felt anything like it in years, of course. It was wonderful! On the
drive home, nothing seemed as I had remembered it and
I wondered if it was the city or me that had changed? I
soon discovered that we had probably both grown.
Melbourne seemed to have had a facelift in my absence.
It seemed so much bigger than I remembered.

**

My family had moved house since I had left for Canada in 1996. My Mum knew it would be really hard for me to go back to the house where I had so many bad experiences and memories. It was also the house that my Mum and Dad had mortgaged to the hilt to help pay for my treatment at Montreux. This financial sacrifice has caused me a great deal of guilt even though my parents say I have nothing to feel guilty about and that they would do it all again to save my life.

Mum, Dad, James, Sam and our three little dogs were living in a two-bedroom townhouse when I came home. This was only temporary while they built a house big enough for all of us to live in, when I eventually came home permanently. For this trip my bedroom was the lounge room, which I loved. I spent my first day shopping, what else does a 21-year-old girl do? I think I spent most of my trip home, apart from rediscovering the beach and re-connecting with my family, cruising the shopping strips of Melbourne in awe of how things had changed.

The first weekend home was consumed with organising my twenty-first birthday party. I know, it was March, and my birthday was in January so it felt a little strange organising a party that was really a farce. I say farce as it was to be filmed by a Channel Nine camera crew for the final instalment in their documentary so we all had to pretend it was actually my twenty-first. In fact, this was to be my fourth twenty-first birthday party. My first was in Canada with friends from Montreux, the second was in California on my actual birthday and the third one was in Utah with my aunt so I was a little partied out by the time it came to do it all again for the cameras. As most of my friends had drifted away over the years I was sick, I really didn't have that many people to invite. I had aunties, uncles, cousins, grandparents, siblings, parents and family friends, all the usual suspects for such an occasion, but it made me feel like a fraud when my brothers and sister had to invite their friends to boost the numbers.

I chose the flowers and a very crazy two-tiered chocolate cake decorated with white chocolate flowers, encrusted in primary coloured jewels bursting out from the centre on long stems. I ate a piece of cake with the feeling that most people in the room were secretly staring at me, especially those who hadn't seen me since I left four years earlier. I wore a blue organza strapless dress. Wearing it in public, not to menton on television, was a huge challenge for me but I didn't give in to any fears that night. I was determined to enjoy myself. We watched embarrassing home movies, another twenty-first must, and I spent most of the night amazed that I had lived to see this day.

I have two favourite moments of that night. The first involved Dad. He didn't want to give a speech but was forced into it as it was sort of his duty. He said I was his hero; a comment that brought a few tears to some of the people at the party. 'Bronte is my hero', those words will linger in my heart forever. Dad explained it like this: 'It was exciting to have Bronte back home. When she went away she wasn't the person we knew. She was a very sick person. Now, the Bronte we knew was back.'

The other moment was dancing with my sister Sam. Everyone had left except for party-all-night Ray Martin and the fun-loving camera crew. We put on a Fatboy Slim CD and cranked up the volume. Sam and I danced around the room to the track 'Praise You', doing the

Fatboy dance from the video clip. We didn't care that all eyes were on us. We let go and danced freely. I hadn't done that in a long, long time.

The day after we had finished filming my twenty-first, my family all got together with Ray and his team for a 'goodbye' lunch. With Ray at the head of the table, I began to reflect on our journey together, as it did really feel like he had been riding beside me on my path to recovery. His genuine passion for my story and the cause was so apparent and has continued to grow. Without Ray's dedication to my story, so many people would still be in the dark about eating disorders. He stood beside my family and me and put a voice and face to the struggle with eating disorders in this country. Ray never wavered in his goal of telling the truth about this horrible illness, always sensitive and protective.

As James was still studying and Sam had just graduated from medicine, they were both still at home. Jordan, now twenty-three had moved out of home and didn't come around very often so I had to seek him out, so to speak. The first substantial amount of time I spent with him was when we went to dinner at a little café on Chapel Street. I will never forget him staring at me as I ate, not moving but just staring in amazement until he finally said, 'I haven't seen you eat in six years.' It was then that I realised it must have felt just as strange for my family having me home as it felt for me being there.

I came home for a visit that was supposed to last just two weeks but enjoyed my time so much that I stayed for a month. The idea of the visit was to test myself and, in a way, test my family to see if we were ready for each other. I discovered I was capable of more than I gave myself credit. Having said that, visiting for a few weeks is very different to living somewhere and I knew there was still work I needed to do in Canada so I reluctantly returned to what felt like my adopted country.

In the space of one month I had faced a huge fear and discovered that I did want to go home to discover what life had to offer and start living. The day I flew back to Canada seemed to sneak up on me quickly. I didn't want to leave my family again. I cried all the way back to Canada. I knew I wouldn't be able to stay away for long before I would want, and need, to come back for good.

Friday, 31 March 2000

I've been back in Canada now for a few days. It doesn't feel like I belong here any more after being home. I feel uneasy about life again. I'm torn as to what to do about my future.

Monday, 1 May 2000

I haven't had the easiest time of it lately. I've found the little things in life are getting harder. I've found it so hard to not count calories. I wasn't counting the calories a few months ago, but in the past few weeks I seemed to be slipping back a little, which is extremely hard.

I've also felt the urge to exercise more lately. I only acted on it a few times but the urge was hard to fight. The good news is that I continue to eat.

I plan to leave Victoria in two months time. I'm not

sure where I'll go – I've just got to get away and move on with life. In the meantime, I'm staying in an apartment organised by Montreux, which means I won't have to stay at the clinic. I don't want to be at the clinic because it can be such a negative environment with all those 'sick' people.

Tuesday, 2 May 2000

I haven't written about my trip to Australia, so here goes. It was mighty hot there despite it being autumn. I had a great time. I spent time with my family, which was fantastic. We went to Brighton Beach and ate out a LOT! We went down the coast to Sorrento and had fish and chips on the beach. We went to the city on the train. We visited Nanna and Poppa Cullis and had dinner with them. We also had dinner with Nanny.

Went out dancing with Jordan at a club on Chapel Street – a street frequently visited as I shopped lots. I ate out for breakfast every Saturday. In fact, I must have tried just about every good restaurant in Melbourne.

Channel Nine organised for me to meet John Farnham, which was an awesome experience. I got to hang out with him and his band and I got to listen to the rehearsal for his new album. I had a very fun day.

We went to look at the new house, which will be exciting when it's finished. We also went to Sydney, had dinner quite a few times and explored the botanic gardens and the art gallery. Oh, and we did more shopping!

I climbed the Sydney Harbour Bridge at night, which was incredible. Next morning I flew to Brisbane with Mum while Dad went home. We went to Sea World and then drove down to Byron Bay. Byron Bay is so beautiful.

After Byron Bay, we flew back to Melbourne and then I flew back to Victoria, Canada about four days later.

Friday, 12 May 2000

I need to keep testing myself to see if I'm really getting better so I'm going to see our relatives in Utah. It'll be great to catch up and to get away from Montreux again as I feel alone here.

Life in Canada wasn't the same after my trip to Australia as I didn't know where I belonged any more. In June 2000 I decided to stay with some of my extended family in America. It seemed like a good step between Canada and going home. I wasn't in my safety zone but I was only a few hours flight away from Montreux if I needed it. I stayed for a month and then returned to Canada.

By this time the Canadian licensing authorities had closed the clinic so I was discharged and moved into an apartment in a nearby suburb. Many of my good friends had gone home and I found myself very alone. I didn't see Peggy or Nicole very much and as I couldn't work, study or volunteer, I became somewhat of a recluse, which wasn't healthy for me. I spent much of this time on the phone to Mum in tears. So Mum being Mum immediately flew over, packed me up and booked a ticket home. I told Peggy and Nicole and their response was not good. They felt I wasn't ready to leave yet and told me that I would be back on their doorstep in three months needing help. I knew it was time for me to return home though.

Saturday, 3 June 2000

I'm back in Victoria, Canada, after my trip to America. It's the start of summer yet it's overcast and cold outside. I'm determined to make my time in Canada better this time. Knowing I'll only be here for a short time before going back to Australia helps me get through the days.

Sunday, 16 July 2000

As I sit here, savouring each bite of my Cherry Ripe, listening to the crash of the ocean waves and with the sun gently beating down on me, all I can think about is . . . everything. My thoughts are all so muddled. There are so many things I need and want to say but I don't think anyone here in Victoria understands me these days.

Thursday, 20 July 2000

I have no education. I have a dull personality and I irritate myself. I'm ugly. But I am the way I am. I feel like I have no purpose here or anywhere. I feel like I don't belong anywhere right now. I don't know where I will be safe any more. By safe I mean safe inside myself.

I feel like I'm only safe in Victoria and I don't want to feel like this is the only safe place for me. I want to feel safe at home, too. I want to know that I can never get sick again. That being sick is NOT A POSSIBILITY. I want and need to move on with my life.

I don't get out of bed until about 2 p.m. and I don't

usually get dressed until 5 p.m. or 6 p.m. This is no life for me. I have BIG dreams and BIG GOALS. But I have no education, and I feel like I'm just wasting time here.

Friday, 21 July 2000

Here's a breakthrough for me – I've been riding the bus just about everywhere. So I'm overcoming my fear of dirt, germs and public spaces. I'm more independent too. I grocery shop for myself and pay the rent. But it's kind of unrealistic in a sense because I'm not working and I don't have any money. I have to rely on Mum and Dad for money, which doesn't feel too independent at all. I'm so torn and so angry inside.

Saturday, 22 July 2000

I'm kind of angry, well annoyed, with Peggy and Nicole. They told me they would keep me busy, spend time with me and help me out a little. I've seen Peggy once and Nicole, well, she's pregnant so I understand she's busy. Sometimes they're so full of it. I don't believe them half the time. I feel so alone all the time. I hate living alone. HATE IT.

Sunday, 23 July 2000

It's sunny and beautiful today, summer at last. It's good to be alive on days like these. It is Sunday, early evening. I came down to the beach to write in my diary. I think it's a good Sunday thing to do.

There's a lot I have to be sorry for, I'm so sorry, it weighs heavily on my heart and I am constantly striving to be better.

A cool breeze is starting to come in, or maybe it's

just because I'm by the water. As I sit and look over at the Olympic Mountains it's hard to comprehend the beauty. What a view. In this very moment I'm lucky, and so blessed that I'm alive to see it.

Tuesday, 25 July 2000

It's late and I've just dropped all the stuff I couldn't fit in my cases at Bill's house to store. I thought about shipping them home but I figure I'll come back to visit soonish, so I'll pick it up then. It's so nice of Bill to look after all my stuff for me. It's amazing really how many possessions one can accumulate in four years.

I had a meeting with Peggy today to catch up before I left. Peggy said the only way I could go home and be safe was if I had constant contact with her and Nicole. She told me of her 'five-year follow-up program' to reduce the risk of relapse. This made me feel a little better but I had a feeling deep inside that the follow-up program wouldn't happen for me.

I'm having lunch with Nicole tomorrow before I catch my plane in Vancouver. I can't believe I'm leaving for good. This is it. I'm not sure how I feel right now.

There were no banners, no balloons and no welcoming committee when I arrived home the second time, the time that I would stay for good. It was now about four months since my visit home. Late July 2000 and Australia was in pre-Olympics mode. Mum and Dad were picking me up at Melbourne airport but in true Clarke style (Mum's genes), they were late. No one seemed too excited that

I was back to stay and I felt a pang of sadness realising life hadn't stopped while I was in Canada. There I was standing with all that I owned in two suitcases staring life in the face. I felt very alone.

I felt like a foreigner in a strange country and strange world. I even felt like a foreigner in my own home and family. I very quickly had to learn how to be a part of a family unit for the first time since I was fifteen. I was now twenty-one. I didn't have much of an education because I left school halfway through Year 10. I had no friends, I didn't have a job and I couldn't see why anyone would employ someone with no experience. To be honest, life seemed pretty bleak and I had an awful thought that this was what I had fought so hard for. I felt trapped in a hopeless world and my new-found circumstances gave me perfect ammunition to convince myself that I was a loser. I felt so far behind everyone else my age. I couldn't see how I could possibly catch up. I became very depressed and things that were much easier for me before I came home suddenly became so much harder. Eating was just one of these things and I lost quite a bit of weight.

I saw a GP about my weight loss, which turned out to be a bit of a turning point for me. We figured out a plan to get me back on track and he turned out to be a great person to talk with, as he seemed to understand the mindset of anorexia extremely well. With the incredible support from my family I began to challenge the many fears that I was only just starting to conquer. I still had a lot of issues with food and being around 'normal' people was helpful in understanding that my behaviours and relationships with food, although much better, were not 'normal'. Being the stubborn person I am, I never gave up. If I was avoiding a situation, whether it be with food or a social interaction I would always ask myself why I was avoiding it. If it was anorexia driven, I would make sure I followed through with the issue no matter how hard it was.

Friday, 15 September 2000

I've just heard the clinic officially closed the other day. I'm so angry and upset about it. But I know that Montreux has not died. The legacy will live on, as will the hope. Just because the building is gone doesn't mean the work will stop.

A Canadian medical inquiry first ordered Montreux to close on 31 January 2000. The clinic was found to have breached a number of Canadian licensing laws. Peggy was allowed to continue Montreux as an out-patient centre while an appeal was heard. She lost the appeal in September 2000 and was forced to close Montreux's doors. Today, Peggy is involved in educating health professionals about eating disorders.

Wednesday, 11 October 2000

Well, it has been too long since I've written in my diary. A lot has happened since I last wrote.

So, here I am in Melbourne. I have been home for about two months. Some weeks have been horrible, others good. Some days have been shocking, others great.

I've been figuring out what to do with my life over the next little while. I had to write a resumé and start a job hunt, which was horrible. After many tears and depressive moments, I ended up getting the first job

I applied for. I got a casual position at the Chadstone
David Jones store in the toy department. I'm very
excited about it and the customers have been really
nice to me. Some seem to recognise me because of my
television appearances. I'm planning to go back to
school next year.

I applied for jobs thinking the entire time that I was a
fool for trying and much to my surprise was offered the
very first job I applied for. I was a Christmas casual in the
toy department at David Jones in Chadstone. I loved it as
it gave me confidence and I discovered many things that
I was good at. The job also gave me the opportunity to
interact with all sorts of people and build new friendships. I felt I was different to everyone else as I got upset
so easily and could see that I was really quite frail in
terms of life experience and my sensitivity. I had to work
so incredibly hard to stay afloat and to try to believe that
everything that went wrong wasn't my fault. I had to
teach myself that I wasn't a bad person and that I
deserved to be on this Earth, just like everyone else.

While I don't have the voice in my head like I used to,
I still have the very occasional, and terrible, moments of
self-doubt. Recently Mum and I were talking about a
series of conversations we had after I applied for the part-
time job when I came home from Canada. Actually, it
was more how my negative mind worked hard to take me
out of play. Paraphrased, it went something like this:

Bronte: I want to apply for a job at David Jones but
what's the point I have nothing to offer? What would
I write in a letter, that I've been sick and in Canada for
the past four years?

Mum: Send in the application anyway. The worst outcome would be that you don't get an interview.
Outcome: I applied and got an interview.

Bronte: I'm going to be found out at the interview. They will never give me the job. I won't turn up.
Mum: Go to the interview, it will give you experience. Many others will also be applying for work. Not everyone will be successful. This doesn't mean they're failures.
Outcome: I went to the interview.

Bronte: I really stuffed that up. They hated me. I'm never going to an interview again.
Mum: You have no proof whatsoever that the interview went badly. In fact, have you even considered that it went well? Notice how 'Neg' always prepares you for failure. What if you have succeeded?
Outcome: I was offered the job.

Bronte: When I start work they'll notice how hopeless I am and I'll be sacked. I should quit now to save the humiliation later.
Mum: DJs are expecting that you'll need training and won't expect you to do and know everything. Allow yourself time to learn.
Outcome: I started the job and was given training.

Bronte: This job is only over Christmas. They'll get rid of me after that. I'm not good enough to keep on.
Mum: Have work said anything to you about not continuing? Why do you listen to 'Neg' without considering that he might be wrong? Why can't you ever consider that things might work out well for you?

Outcome: I was offered ongoing employment.

Bronte: Everyone at DJs has a service star. I'll never get one because I'm so hopeless.
Outcome: I was awarded not only a service star but also a special award for legendary service.

Bronte: They only gave me that because they feel sorry for me because I'm such a loser.

At this point Mum sat me down and pointed out that no matter what I wanted to do in life, 'Neg' would try to protect me from the risk of failure by making me give up and hide. She helped me see this is what my anorexia was all about.

I can't really remember who gave my negative mind the name 'Neg' but I think it was Mum. Naming the negative mind helped me recognise these thoughts as a bully at work and it gave me strength to fight the illness. This is something that really helps me. It's a relief to know that the unrealistic ideals, the haughtiness, the expectations, the self-loathing, hatred and the saboteur within are not me. These are the opposite of what I'm striving to achieve in life. I know this now because I can separate 'Neg' the voice from me. I can then retaliate.

When I was sick, I was not expected to do the things normally expected of a young person. Even though my life was torture, I couldn't try to make things better in case I failed and embarrassed myself. Not failing meant that I would not disappoint or let anyone down. In fact, 'Neg' made me feel successful in one way. I was very, very good at starving! This is one area of my life where I reached the top. The only problem was that it was 'Neg's' achievement, not mine. 'Neg's' crowning glory would have been my death. I know that now, but when I was trapped within 'Neg's' control, I couldn't see the risk to my life. Perhaps this is why anorexia is such a life-threatening illness. At the point where you need to see the truth, it is hidden away by the negative thoughts.

I have moments when I wish that not so many people knew I was anorexic because of television. It's something people judge you on before they get to know you. I can't hide my past, nor do I want to. Having said that, I don't regret the television experience because it's also helped to make me who I am. I've met some amazing people along the way and I continue to. It also means I can help people. I feel it's important otherwise what's the point of life? Perhaps the whole media thing was meant to happen.

Being recognised in public makes me feel awkward. Sometimes when people say, 'You're Bronte, aren't you?' I feel like answering, 'No I'm not.' I remember shopping at Myer one day when a woman came up to me and said, 'Sorry, I have to interrupt you. I'm a Home Economics teacher and we watch videos on you at school and I just think you're so fantastic and an inspiration.' Another time, I was with a friend in a shop in Melbourne's Botanic Gardens. My friend said, 'Bronte, look at this.' The salesperson, who would have been in her 60s, turned around and said, 'Bronte? Our Bronte? Is that our Bronte, the one with anorexia?' She asked how I was and what I was doing. The interest is lovely and touching but it's also awkward because I don't know these people. I always thank them for their interest but I always ask them their name and ask how they are.

I met a lot of really good customers while working at David Jones. Back in 2000, I had people coming up to me all the time having seen me on Channel Nine. People say, 'There's something about you that is just different and it's really compelling. It's not even about your illness, it's just about you.' I don't take compliments very well, especially when I don't think so highly of myself.

When people say these things or write to say how I've helped them that's when I think, 'Wow, that's pretty fabulous that I could help one person.' After all, that's all I ever wanted to do. I think there's a part of me that's a bit of a crusader, like Mum, that thinks people need to know what this disease is about. I remember reading about the anorexic Kendall twins from London and thinking why doesn't someone just make them eat? But it's not until you're in that situation that you can understand what they're going through in terms of anorexia. On one level I could understand their mindset but I didn't know what anorexia was all about.

In the end the entire media experience has been a bit of a double-edged sword for me. I have met some of the most incredible people and I have discovered and built great friendships that I treasure dearly. Through the media I have discovered the goodness of humanity and my family and I have received letters of encouragement, love, friendship and financial support from families and individuals from around Australia who I don't even know. I've been completely blown away by the kindness of the public. It is a relief to know such beauty, kindness and love still exists in a world that seems so damaged by evil most of the time. With the help of the media, albeit hard to understand at times, I've been able to help those who want to learn and know what a day in the life of an eating disorder sufferer is like and what the condition is really about.

Friday, 13 October 2000

I've been busy helping Sam get ready for her wedding next March. She has picked her dress and she looks beautiful in it. She's heading off to Traralgon in country Victoria for three months to work as a resident doctor. I'm missing her already even though she likes to pick fights with me every now and then. She is a good sister. Jordan is still cold towards me. I guess it will take some time to heal the deep emotional wounds. I just want to see everyone happy.

Well, it's time to go now. I have a dog next to me who is itching to go for a walk. Come to think of it, I feel like a walk also. It's nice to finally be free . . . free to walk in the sunshine. Free. Just me and my dog Bob.

Bye.

The Montreux Clinic rarely contacted me after my return home. It was quite a hurtful reality that perhaps I wasn't worth keeping in touch with. Three months came and went and I wasn't knocking on their door for help. I began to see my family as an important group of people who wanted to help me and wouldn't allow me to get sick again. To my surprise they understood me far more than I had given them credit and I began to trust them with so many of my fears. It got to the point they knew what was going on in my head before I even said it out loud. They became, and continue to be, an unbelievable support for me. I know that I wouldn't be where I am if I didn't have them.

From where I sit, Canada seems like a lifetime ago. I felt homesick for my island hideaway of Victoria for a while but, as time passed, Australia became my home once again. I see it as a completely different place to the one I left on a cold April day in 1996.

2001

In 2001, eight months after my return to Australia I received a phone call at 2 a.m. and I knew something was wrong. It was a counsellor from the Montreux Clinic telling me that my dear friend Becca had died in her sleep at home. Her mum had gone to wake her in the morning to find her not breathing. I had only spoken to Becca a month before trying to encourage her to want to live, to hang on. I felt such frustration, almost anger, at her for giving up but by this stage she was completely consumed by her anorexia and there was not much of Becca left.

That was my last conversation with her. I didn't tell her how much I loved her and how I would always cherish her friendship. I didn't tell her that this world would have lost one of the things that made it great if she let anorexia kill her. I didn't share these thoughts, just my frustration. I wish I could have that conversation over again. She was barely twenty-one.

Becca wanted to become a paediatrician and help kids. She wanted to fall in love, marry and have kids of her own one day. She wanted freedom from the condition that had consumed her for half her life. It breaks my heart that she never reached her potential, that others didn't get to share in her life and inner beauty the way I did at her 'good' times. She died alone with no support, except that of her mum and dad. If she had been a child with cancer there would have been sufficient support groups for her family to help them deal with her life and death. There would have been support and love for her from society, and efforts would have been made to 'enrich her last days on Earth'. Why did Becca, who died from a psychological illness, deserve less than someone who dies from a physical illness? I miss her. I not only live for me but I live for her.

Anorexia kills. This is a reality and it is why, although terribly hard and raw at times, I'm involved in helping others today.

I started checking out possibilities for study in 2001. I mainly looked at fine arts but became rather flat when I soon realised that almost everything I wanted to do required a Victorian Certificate of Education (VCE) in English. Despite this hurdle, I decided on a course I thought I would enjoy and applied thinking there was no way I could get in. I was wrong, again, and in March I started my Certificate IV in Arts in make-up design at Swinburne University in Melbourne. I discovered it was something I was very good at and enjoyed but it was also a challenge to be so sensitive among a group of women who could be very competitive and very bitchy. And through my experiences with David Jones and study, I was beginning to learn that there is a lot of nastiness in the world and that not everyone you meet will like you or you them.

I had many days of tears, anger and frustration at who I was, hating the fact that I was so sensitive. I felt I was so dumb compared to the rest of the world and found it very hard to acknowledge any talent I had. It felt like

I had enrolled in a crash course in life and I was having to experience and live all the things most people do over a decade in just one year. It was extremely overwhelming and at times I felt I just couldn't cope and that maybe I just wasn't meant to be a part of this world.

In 2002, I began a two year diploma in interior decoration and design that I have just finished. Again, along with learning about interior design, it became a learning experience for life. There were many times I wanted to quit when I thought I was hopeless and would never be smart enough to complete the course. I had to deal with the issues of relating to competitive girls my age, a situation they had all gone through in high school but one that I had yet to experience.

I had to learn to be stronger and bigger than them and to not let others dictate my worth. I had to learn to deal with people that I clashed with but I also came to the understanding that it's not bad to be an individual. I realised that I was glad that I didn't fit in with the clique of girls my age who seemed to behave like sheep following a leader. I was glad that I had my own thoughts and ideas and I was proud that I didn't feel the need to conform and that my ethics and values never wavered. Having said that, it's not easy feeling there aren't many people you can relate to. At times it seems very lonely because of this. I have been lucky that I have found similar souls along the way and it is these people and relationships that make the world a nicer place.

Part Five

Why Me?

After months of living with anorexia I began to think: why me? Why is this happening to me? It's not that I would wish it on anyone else but rather I didn't want to be suffering this way. Who would? I really didn't understand what anorexia was or why I was its victim. The only answer I could come up with was that I deserved this illness because I was such a bad person.

I now know that anorexia didn't choose me nor did I choose it. I was predisposed to anorexia. I was born with a negative mindset and I was developing anorexia all my life as my negative mind got stronger. So why was I predisposed and not my brothers and sister? I have asked myself this question many times and the answer is simple.

My mother tells me that I was the most imaginative, most creative and by far the most sensitive of all her children. I was a sensitive child, just as I will always be a sensitive adult. I'm more aware of that sensitivity now and I'm learning how to channel it in a positive direction rather than a negative one. I'm learning that other people's problems are outside my circle of control and that it's not my responsibility to fix these problems, even if I feel I should. I'm learning how to listen to others and to trust what they tell me rather than listen to the inner critic who leads me towards self-loathing. I have learned to switch off from the overwhelming negative voice of the world news, for the most part. To switch off the despair that I can't change.

While I was predisposed to anorexia and always hypersensitive as a child, there were three major events, triggers, as I call them, in my life that probably set off my illness and go right back to my childhood. I suffered at the brutal hands of bullies at school, I suddenly lost an important childhood friendship and my Nanny almost died.

I was a highly sensitive 11-year-old girl and I was bullied mercilessly at school in Rowville. The bullying happened day in, day out. I would arrive home in tears everyday and go to school late each day. I would avoid school by using every tactic known to me. It wasn't as if there were just one or two bullies. It was a whole group of kids known as the 'cool lovers gang' which was con-doned by my teacher who thought the gang was cute. This was such a tumultuous and painful year for me and by the time my parents moved me to another school after the first term of Year 6, I had retreated into my shell and never felt safe to come out again. My negative mind finally had evidence that people didn't like me, that I was a lesser person than others and that I would never fit in. The bullet was in the chamber, waiting to be fired.

During the first months of school, Mum would re-assure me that the other children were just jealous, to stand tall and not give in. Mum would give different advice today. Mum appealed to the teacher and school but it all fell on deaf ears. Not knowing what else to do, other than build me up, Mum sent me back where the bullies finished me off. By end of first term Mum knew that if she didn't get me out of there, those children, and the refusal of the school to see what was happening, would kill me.

Mum arranged for me to be transferred to the school where she taught. It was a drastic act to remove a child halfway through their final year of primary school but Mum and Dad had to do something. My new teacher, Margaret Addison, was kind and wonderful but it wasn't enough to undo the damage that had already been done. My new classmates were viewed with caution; potential bullies loomed all around. This was the beginning of the end for me.

High school, although somewhat of a relief after primary school, was another enormous toxic change for me. I went to an all-girls school in a quiet inner-city suburb of Melbourne. It was quite a distance from my house, which meant it would take the best part of 2 hours to travel to school and back each day. Girls, as I knew, could be very bitchy so, feeling frightened of not fitting in, I alienated myself. My reasoning was that if I was inaccessible to others, then I couldn't be rejected. I cried just about every day because I felt like I didn't have friends and that no one liked me. I struggled with the work. My school reports always said, 'Bronte would do so well if she actually put in the effort.' But I always thought, 'Well, why bother because I'm just stupid anyway.' When I started to get sick I used to hide in the corner of the classroom and sleep. I wasn't even listening any more, I would put my head on the table and go to sleep. At school I was always afraid that even if I did try I would fail and that would really mean that I was more stupid than I thought I was, if that was possible.

The second trigger was the sudden disappearance of

my very good friend, Rachel. As I explained earlier, Rachel was the one person who understood me at school. We were very close and then one day she was gone. She never said goodbye. I thought it was my fault. I thought it was impossible for anyone to like or understand me. This was a pivotal moment and, coupled with my self-loathing and sensitivity, became the point when the gun's safety latch was removed.

Not long after Rachel vanished came the third trigger. As I've mentioned, doctors discovered that Nanny had a tumour in the right side of her face. She was admitted to St Vincent's Hospital in central Melbourne for surgery. It was all too much for me at this point. She was one of my best friends. She sat by my bed when I was a baby fighting for my life. I felt I owed her my life, the thought of losing her was lethal. My Nanny's illness pulled the final trigger. I stopped eating. Three weeks later I was admitted to hospital and life was never the same again.

Part Six

Am I Cured?

Life can be so beautiful. As I sit here and reflect on my life I feel so blessed that I have sight to see the beauty and wonders that surround me. I'm on top of a hill overlooking the Pacific Ocean and I'm close enough to hear the sound of the waves crashing on the beach below. The air smells sweet and the gum trees seem to have a greater depth of colour and richness to them. I feel I could live in this moment forever and feel complete contentment. It feels as if there's no one else on Earth but this natural beauty, my family and good friends surrounding me. Oh, if only life were this simple more often.

So here I sit enjoying the beauty that I might never have been able to see, feel or enjoy had I not been strong enough, and had the support, to get to this point today. It's very confronting and it hurts to open old wounds by re-living and writing about my journey but I've also been reminded of the pivotal lessons these experiences have taught me – never feel you've lost a race when you haven't even begun running it and recognise the importance of faith, belief and trust. Without these things we would all live in an utter state of hopelessness. Nothing would seem worthwhile.

There's a misconception about anorexia and the process of recovery. There seems to be this idea that most people have that if you look better now and can eat, you're cured. This is so WRONG.

This illness not only robbed me of the 'the best years of my life' but it also stole my sense of self, my self-esteem. Yes, I can eat and like every other woman on this planet I have body issues. Perhaps I feel the 'fat days' a little more intensely and more often than others but I don't allow these fears to get out of control to the point where I begin starving myself again. I know that in order to enjoy a 'Good quality of life', to be able to study, swim, socialise, travel, paint, design, have kids and grow old, I need to be a 'normal body weight' for my height. Yes, I have days when I know I'm not seeing myself correctly, when my perception is clearly warped. But in order to recover emotionally, I also had to recover physically and vice-versa. As I continue to re-enter life, many things have become more important than my weight. What's important is how I feel inside, my relationships with others, my boyfriend, my family, my hopes and dreams, and the reality of all these things coming to fruition. I want to continue living to see where life takes me.

I'm often asked what my lowest weight was, even though you can't judge how sick an anorexic is by how much he or she weighs. I don't really remember what my lowest weight was, I think it was 38 kilograms. When I got sick I had a goal weight of 37 kilograms. I don't know why my condition chose that weight. As I got closer to this goal weight it dawned on me that it wasn't low enough and a new goal weight was set. This was a perpetual cycle. It would never have been low enough until it was zero. It used to make me so angry that my parents were so intent on keeping me alive.

I'm ever so grateful that I have a healthy body now, that I'm not riddled with osteoporosis, that I don't have any organ damage and that I'll be able to have children one day. Sadly these are unattainable luxuries for many recovering victims of an eating disorder. I feel lucky everyday that the abuse my body suffered was not permanent.

I don't know what my weight is today. I haven't known a number since I set foot on Canadian soil almost eight years ago. I don't want to know what it is. A number doesn't define who I am, nor does it dictate my worth. I'm so aware of how that nasty negative mind of mine works and how it would take that number and give it more importance and status than it deserves. I now use the tools and strength I have acquired over the years of battle to protect myself. This is not to say I'll never know my weight. Maybe one day I will find out by default and again it will be another challenge along my road of recovery.

I did go through a period of gaining weight. I hadn't been eating anything different so my instant reaction was, 'This is out of control. I should stop eating.' Mum helped me see the reason why it was happening and that reverting to old anorexia coping mechanisms would not help the situation in the long run. I knew she was right. I knew if I stopped eating, or restricted my food intake, I would create an opening and an opportunity for my negative mind to gain more control and escape the little box I had him locked up in.

I decided to see a dietician and together we discovered that I was going through puberty at twenty-four! My whole body shape changed. My skin changed and I grew breasts for heaven's sake . . . I was horrified. It was all very hard to deal with but I took these changes as more challenges and obstacles to soldier through. My old instinct was to retreat to a safe place inside myself. But as I've said, life was far too interesting and promising to give up on when I'd come this far. So I said to myself that these changes too shall pass and everyone around me assured me that my body would find its comfortable place and that the weight gain would stop. I held onto their words with blind faith and, instead of slipping back, I forged on to discover my family were right and my body shape and weight settled down.

Everyone started commenting on how good I looked which made me angry. Good means fat to the negative mind. My family kept reassuring me that I wasn't big but that I looked beautiful and healthy and didn't look anorexic any more. I now looked like a woman. This was so hard to hear because in a way I was letting go of all that I'd known for so long.

Now that we have the 'body', or exterior of the house, covered let's move onto the interior structure. The self. Life certainly hasn't been easy since returning home with an expectation from society that goes something like this, 'The only people we accept in this world are other people like us. We don't like people who are different, who may need a different approach. We view them as weak, we don't like people we don't understand as we're afraid of things we can't comprehend and we are, in general, too arrogant, too ignorant and self-absorbed to even bother trying. If you don't fit with what we consider normal we don't want you around'. I've been made to feel like I'm wrong rather than a result of society's ignorance and intolerance. This simply compounded everything negative that I felt about myself and is probably one of the very reasons I got sick in the first place. Having to learn to survive in this world without being engulfed in the tentacles of anorexia again has been one of the hardest things to endure. There have been so many moments when I've wanted to give up but I take a breath, look around and think about all the reasons to keep going. It's been a bloody hard road to get to where I am today, but I'm defiant and strong and I'm not going to give up life for anything.

Am I cured? I know this is the question on the tip of your tongue. I imagine it has been since you started reading. I can eat almost anything. I write 'almost' because like you, I've rediscovered my likes and dislikes and can honestly say that I avoid certain foods, not because I'm afraid of them, but rather because I simply don't like the taste or texture.

I don't, however, feel complete freedom within myself. I can't always see my good qualities and talents, although I seem to find it very easy to find bad ones. This is something I'm getting better at with more practise at life.

I have intense feelings that can be both positive and negative. I tend to take everything said to me far more personally than it was meant and over-analyse things. I find this very frustrating.

I'm often plagued with the feeling and urge to gather up everyone's problems, stresses and troubles and solve them. I feel different to others my age and I often feel misunderstood.

My sensitivity is misinterpreted as snobbishness when really all I want is to feel accepted for who I am. I say sorry all the time for things that aren't my fault. I have days when I loathe myself, when I hate my reflection.

I have days when I feel I will never be right for the world. I have days when I think everyone hates me, that I'm a burden to my family and society and that life won't get easier.

Despite all of that, I do have days and moments of pure joy and laughter, freedom and happiness as well as days of acknowledgment that I'm not as bad as I seem. Life continues to get better. As I gain more life experience, the bright days take over from my days of despair and as time goes by I grow stronger inside. I'm discovering who I am after so many years of being lost inside a world of anorexia. Recovery from an eating disorder is similar to how I imagine a former alcoholic and drug addict must feel. It's something that I will always have to keep in check. I can't go on a crazy fad diet and not expect it to get out of hand. Anorexia is not something that consumes me as it did in the past and I'm free from its grasp. Recovery is possible.

Epilogue

There was a time, at age fifteen, when I didn't think I would be alive to see my eighteenth birthday. I'm now twenty-five and I've defied the odds. I can't focus on the past. I can't regain my lost years and experiences but what I can do is live to the full every day of my future. I have a blank canvas before me. Every stroke of paint I add is part of my continual journey of life and recovery. I know that life will be rocky but it's only through the bitter that I can taste the sweet. It is for those sweet moments that I live for.

I want to experience the world from every angle. I want to live life, step outside my comfort zone and discover what is around me. I want to discover my country, other countries and cultures. I want to discover the universal language of the world that sets us apart yet brings us together – humanity. I want to study more. I hope that I never stop learning. I want to work to live, not the other way around. I hope that I never neglect my passion and talents and I will paint and create and help others until I'm old and grey. I want to be able to say at the end of my life, 'I made a difference in the world. I brought about change and paved a way of understanding for the next generation so that they don't suffer the way I did'.

Am I in love? The answer is yes, and it warms me to know he is beside me in all that I do. I wish I could give

you a fairytale ending, tell you there will be marriage and
children, that I will one day find inner peace and quiet
and with this a contentment and love for myself, but I
don't know that, yet. These are my hopes and dreams.
I wish I knew the answers. Unfortunately nobody knows
the future, but anything is possible.

This I do know.

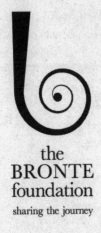

the
BRONTE
foundation
sharing the journey

For those needing support and treatment for eating disorders, please contact the Bronte Foundation at www.thebrontefoundation.com.au.